REPEAT PRESCRIPTION

More Riotous Stories from the
Country Practice

Also available

Country Doctor
*Hilarious True Stories from
a Country Practice*

REPEAT PRESCRIPTION

More Riotous Stories from the Country Practice

ROBINSON
London

Constable & Robinson Ltd
3 The Lanchesters
162 Fulham Palace Road
London W6 9ER
www.constablerobinson.com

First published in the UK by Robinson,
an imprint of Constable & Robinson, 2004

A copy of the British Library Cataloguing in
Publication Data is available from the British Library

ISBN: 978-1-78033-052-5

Printed and bound in the EU

3 5 7 9 10 8 6 4 2

For Teresa, Natalia and Archie

. . . and in memory of my friend John Pitchford, who died whilst on holiday in Australia in February 2003 and must surely have earned his own mention in the book of 'Famous Last Words'.

'I wish I could stop coughing,' he said to his wife, Margot, and sadly – he did . . .

With thanks to my dedicated, committed, supportive . . . well, my staff, anyway, in (hopefully) chronological order – Jenny, Chris, Mandy, Karen, Tessa, Debbie, Lesley, Alison and Jo, for muddling along as best they can through both the difficult times, and the very difficult ones.

My thanks also to the un-named member of the Launceston Camera Club, who – if I had ever needed it – helped me keep my feet firmly on the ground.

When asked by my friend Jon Hicks if he would like a signed copy of my first book he merely grunted, 'Huh – can't get a ruddy appointment with him any time now, he's too busy doing bloody interviews.'

'I'll put you down as a maybe, then Jon, shall I?'

Contents

Introduction   1

1 Setting the Scene   6

2 Anything for a Bet   28

3 A Spell in Casualty   52

4 Doctors, Dentists and Bob   82

5 Little Men with Big Egos – and Vice Versa   104

6 Headley and St Mawgan   124

7 Wroughton, and a Little Problem with . . . Fletch   140

8 The End Game   177

9 Lifton – the Early Years   184

10 Finding my Feet   213

11 We Thought it was All Over . . .   236

12 Exercising My . . .   262

13 Walking the Tightrope   283

Introduction

There are today, as I am sure we would all agree, a whole host of excellent and exceptionally detailed tourist guides for any traveller visiting exotic locations around the world. Take your choice – Namibia, Montenegro, South America . . . Eurodisney, Bognor Regis and yes, even you, Mrs Irene Stapleton at Number 43 Stamford Drive, Blackpool – all of them comprehensively catered for and expounded upon in the greatest detail.

The list is endless, but nowhere – as I have recently discovered after a lengthy and exhaustive investigation – is the one beacon of light that all my devoted readers have been most in need of.

How neglected the three of you have been.

I give you therefore my own indispensable contribution to the uncharted territories of the scarily unknown universe, namely:

THE TRAVELLER'S GUIDE TO VISITING YOUR GP

It can be a traumatic affair, consulting your local doctor – sometimes even for the patients, as well. Here are a few tips on how to survive.

1. Making an appointment

Try to book well in advance – before you are ill, preferably. If however that is impractical then aim to book as late as possible, by which time you will have hopefully recovered from the ailment you wanted attending to in the first place. Ninety per cent of all the patients we see would recover without any interference from their GP whatsoever, whilst the remaining ten per cent sadly often have their illnesses prolonged by our intervention.

Observe the daily climatic changes – an unexpectedly sunny day in a long, cold, rainy spell brings all the weak, infirm and terminally unemployed out into the open. What better way to pass the morning than a gentle gossip down at the surgery, wondering what affliction ails the young man in the corner who seems unable to sit down for more than a few moments at a time?

In much the same way a stormy midsummer day draws in the dedicated 'No point in going to the beach, and not a good time to go shopping' malingerers. 'I know,' they nod sagely to each other, 'let's get ourselves down to the doctor's. It's generally warm and dry in there . . .'

Don't whatever you do make the mistake of one of our patients who recently rang demanding an appointment for a time when she wouldn't 'have to wait'. We gave her one just after lunchtime, knowing full well both doctors would be out on their afternoon visits. She subsequently left, thoroughly disgruntled, after sitting alone for an hour in an empty waiting room.

'Well, she didn't have to wait,' I reasoned thoughtfully on my return. 'She could have turned round and gone straight home again.'

2. Arriving at the surgery

Try smiling at the receptionists immediately upon entering the building. They will be so taken aback by this unusual approach that they will help you in any way they can . . . which in many surgeries, including our own, is unfortunately not very much at all.

Always make sure you have dressed appropriately for the consultation – so many of them are videoed for training purposes these days, and would you really want to be caught on film in *that*? And no more than three layers of clothing, please, especially in the depths of winter, and never wear a tight-fitting dress if you need your abdomen examined . . . which applies to all you women out there, as well.

3. *Entering the waiting room*

Look around carefully before choosing your seat.

Avoid positioning yourself next to anyone who catches your eye as you walk in – they will want to talk to you about how painful *their* haemorrhoids are, not yours. Try and gauge who might be interested in your revolutionary approach to chronic nasal discharge.

Examine meticulously the topography of the entire area. If all those patiently waiting are huddled together in one corner of the room whilst one poor soul sits in splendid isolation in another, avoid him or her like the plague. They may have it.

Observe them intently for signs of small insect infestation, and if they are not actively scratching, then you will have your answer. They will almost certainly smell horribly of stale urine, and be staining the seats.

Double check on anyone who appears to be asleep, to make sure they are still breathing.

4. *Consulting your doctor*

Glance surreptitiously at the television on the bookcase immediately upon entering the consulting room to see whether it is switched on. If the volume is fully turned up it is indubitably a bad sign. Be very afraid of consulting doctors such as myself during an English Test Match, the World Cup or any rugby international, unless you are comfortable with profane and abusive language.

Abstain from all extremes of emotion wherever possible. You may occasionally allow yourself a sympathetic smile should your GP make a passing attempt at a joke – we need all the encouragement we can get – but don't for goodness sake ever dissolve into tears. We none of us will know how to cope, and you cannot guarantee all the tissues in the box will be fresh ones – particularly if it is the end of the week.

Try not to anticipate a definitive diagnosis – we deal primarily in 'funny turns', 'viruses' and 'there's a lot of it about' – whatever 'it' may prove to be – and are not generally forthcoming with precise definitions of your ailments unless there is a good laugh to be had somewhere at your expense. I find a good case of scabies cheers me up no end, with a boil on the bum coming a close second.

On a more serious note, don't ever expect your doctor to like you, or be the least bit interested in whatever intriguing combination of rare conditions you might have presented with. We none of us entered the profession for the benefit of our patients, as you must by now realize.

Finally, and by far the most importantly, turn up a good twenty minutes late for your appointment – we won't be running to time, so why on earth should you? Better still, don't bother to turn up at all.

And if you want to make your GP really happy, book an appointment with him you have absolutely no need for, preferably early on a Monday morning, and cancel it five minutes before you are due to arrive. Remember that every doctor who has ever lived hates these unequivocal sessions from hell even more than you do.

Plan then for a further 'conflagration in hell' in a week's time, and later cancel that too. That way, you and your GP can look forward to not meeting each other again, and again, and again . . .

You will therefore be for ever elevated to the ranks of our favourite patients, to whom we send all those unwanted Christmas presents we receive – yes, you've guessed it, the Lambrusco, cheap whisky and sweet sherry – as a sign of our everlasting, undying appreciation.

5. *Leaving the building*

Walk quickly, and don't look back.

1

Setting the Scene

There will be some of you — in fact, to the best of my calculations, a number well in excess of fifty-nine million in the UK alone — who will not have read my first book, *Country Doctor: Tales of a Rural GP*.

This despite the fact that it won the Lifton Golden Circle 'Book of the Fortnight' award and was the best-seller in our village for a whole week — until the local Scouts released their definitive, ground-breaking tome, *Twenty of Your Favourite Campfire Recipes*.

'So how is fame affecting you?' a patient of mine asked the other day.

'Not nearly as much as I hoped it would,' I answered sadly.

'But you must have made loads of money, surely?' he persisted.

'Well, let's put it this way,' I answered, after due consideration. 'Having balanced the truly magnificent royalties I have received against the comparatively minor expenses it has cost me, I must be one of the few authors on earth who was actually given a tax rebate.'

'It's done that well, then,' he said, pulling a face.

'My agent tells me it's like building a wall,' I explained. 'Each book forms a layer of bricks, one upon the other, until you have constructed a solid, dependable structure that will last for all time.'

'So the first book was a sort of foundation stone, then?' he suggested kindly. 'The rock upon which your future career will be based.'

'Sort of,' I agreed. 'Or at least it would have been had it not sunk without trace in the mud at the bottom of the garden . . .'

For those of you therefore unacquainted with my literary efforts – a number growing daily as some of my original readers will no doubt have died by now, and I suspect few of the new generation of babies born since January 2002 will have yet discovered the book's delights – I thought it best to set out in authentic detail the long and painful journey from childhood to my current exalted position as a GP in a village few people have ever heard of and part-time author of books the vast majority of people will never read.

I was born, the sixth son of itinerant gypsies – my father was one of the few people I know who actually ran away from the circus to become a teacher, rather than the other way round – on a grass verge a mile outside Wellingborough, Northants, in May 1957.

Following an exemplary Borstal education – joy-riding and company fraud a speciality – I graduated to St Mary's, Paddington, on the strength of my one major academic achievement to date . . . the cycling proficiency badge (second class). There I hoped to fulfil my dream, live out my vocation by following in my father's footsteps and emerge on the front steps of the college triumphantly waving my teacher training certificate, but there was one small fly in the ointment.

Nobody had told me it was actually a medical school, not a college at all, and to be totally honest, I was never in the building long enough during the course of the next five years to find out. All my dreams were as dust – I had a medical degree (one of the Australian students suddenly decided to embark on a world tour the day after finals, and kindly left his behind for me to make the best use of it I could) but really very little idea what I should be doing with it.

My next year was spent as a junior doctor in NHS hospitals, mostly wandering the corridors late at night looking for the canteen and the nurses' residential accommodation. I then sought refuge in the RAF as a GP trainee, leaving six years later with a little more knowledge under my belt and rather a lot more expensive medical equipment than I had previously possessed in the boot of my car.

For the past fifteen years I have been settled in the West Country, where my patients have finally realized that they must either put up with my unorthodox brand of medicine or move house, possibly for at least another generation.

On my arrival in Devon in 1988 I was lucky enough to inherit a thriving village practice of some 1,800 patients, all eager to meet their new doctor and lend their utmost support as I embarked upon the latest stage of my professional development. Fifteen years later, by dint of my unstinting efforts, I have now whittled the practice down to twenty-three patients and a couple of dogs, most of whom are reconsidering their options.

During the course of my career I have been fortunate enough to travel extensively − Belize, in South America, during the notorious 'Monkey Nut Scandal'; Cape Town, in South Africa, at the height of the unrest over apartheid; Kosovo, in the aftermath of the war; Ethiopia, during the last devastating famine; and Barrow-in-Furness, just after Vickers, the local dockyard, had finally closed down.

As I sit here now at my word processor, looking back over all those weird and wonderful experiences, all those unexplained deaths, my mind is drawn back to where it first started, now more than a quarter of a century ago.

St Mary's Hospital Medical School, Praed Street, Paddington, London, in October 1975. A crowded lecture theatre, an expectant hush, and suddenly we were off, launched headlong into a breathless journey that would never end . . .

'Whatever you do,' said Oscar, hopping from one foot to the other as if he had recently taken up fire-walking and had yet to fully master the art, 'do it with confidence. And for goodness sake, m'dears, try your utmost not to look too stupid when you make a mistake.'

Note the phraseology – not 'if' you make a mistake, but 'when', as inevitably we would. And did.

He had a lot of common sense, did Oscar, which kind of made you wonder how, as a high-flying consultant, he came to be lecturing to us in the first place. I can only conclude – strange though it may seem – that he must have actually enjoyed it.

Oscar was a delightful little Irishman in his late fifties who looked as if he should have been a leprechaun but grew just a little too big, or a jockey but stayed a little too small. He always treated us as if we were his personal confidants rather than a tedious duty to be attended to, which in many respects we must have been. For Oscar, bless his little cotton socks, was the clinical director of the medical school, a role that suited him to a T.

'Shall I be telling you what I did today . . ?' he would begin a lecture, or 'Can you imagine my surprise when . . ?'

I have no idea whether this was a deliberately cultivated approach or not, but either way Oscar had the knack of personalizing medicine, making you feel as if you were sharing an experience with him rather than struggling along in the black pit of your insecurities on your own. With the benefit of hindsight I can now see that this was his way of introducing us to the then unknown concept of holistic medicine. He was trying to teach us how to empathize with the patient in front of us, looking at them as a person in their own right rather than a collection of random signs and symptoms, another statistic, another trolley in the corridor of life with nowhere to go.

It was one of the few things I took from medical school into the outside world that wasn't somebody else's personal property.

But they weren't all like Oscar, more's the pity. There were sadly very few of him around.

We had, for example, a highly intelligent black pharmacology lecturer who I am sure must have taught us something useful, but all I can now remember is the way he continually impressed upon us that he was black – and highly intelligent. Then there was the eminent American professor, who spent so much of his time emphasizing he was American, eminent and a professor that I cannot for the life of me remember what it was that he taught. For biochemistry – a beautiful subject, if ever there were one – we were blessed with Eric 'By-name', whose real surname was Idle. I leave you to work it out for yourselves.

And then there was J.P.R Williams, the phenomenal Wales and British Lion full-back who was such a joy to watch in action on the rugby field – even (through gritted teeth) for an Englishman. He taught us anatomy for a while in the dissection room, or at least, that was the official version. Looked at another way, however, whilst concealing himself in the guise of a lecturer he might just possibly have been quietly learning the anatomy he never absorbed as a student because he was away playing rugby all the time. The medical school hierarchy, disinterested party though they pretended to be and who would never of course admit it, benefited from his continued presence and availability for the most important part of the entire academic calendar – no, not our finals, but the Inter-Hospitals Rugby Cup.

There were various styles of lecturing for us to observe.

The stand-up comedian approach was always a favourite, with our dispenser of knowledge roving the aisles restlessly, microphone in hand, ready at a moment's notice to clip the ear of any student threatening to fall asleep.

'Good afternoon, my name's Paul, and you've been a lovely audience . . .'

Stuck indelibly in my cerebral cortex is the mindless droning of the neurophysiologist who recited textbook descriptions of bits of the brain you had never even heard of and, as a student, were rarely – if ever – likely to use.

Whilst the former approach was educational in its way — it taught you to live on your wits but often gave you little of practical value save for developing the ability to duck quickly and often — the latter could have bored for England, but you got an awfully good set of lecture notes. Of course, you could have simply gone out, bought his book and saved yourself a lot of trouble, but I suspect I would have just used it to swat flies or prop up a wobbly table or two rather than reading it.

The point was, I suppose, that students attended lectures because it was required of them, whereas the lecturers brought along their own agendas. And that, for better or worse, is where I learned it was essential, if I were to aspire to a future life of happiness in the world of medicine, to develop an agenda of my own — preferably one which didn't involve treating patients, if that were at all possible. Over the years it has been fed, and nurtured, ultimately to travel surreptitiously down with me to this woefully deprived neck of . . . sorry, this idyllic backwater of old-fashioned rural life.

For now I have been content to let my agenda slumber in the peace of our surroundings, but one day, one quiet, unassuming mid-week morning, it will rise unexpectedly, as a phoenix from the ashes, to be unleashed with a vengeance on the unsuspecting practice population like the Midwich Cuckoos, but with more attitude.

Tutorials could be fun, though.

The process of establishing where they were actually taking place was always educational, and often randomly controlled. We would start off in the medical school foyer with a map, a compass and a set of totally incomprehensible directions, almost inevitably written in some sort of Egyptian hieroglyphics. At a given signal — generally an exasperated announcement over the medical school Tannoy that 'Year Two' was in danger of collective expulsion, again, unless somebody somewhere turned up to something they were expected to be at within the next few moments – off we would go, in search of our mystical destination like the Knights of the Round Table in their unending quest for the Holy Grail. This would routinely involve visiting parts of the medical school and the hospital – and very often quite a lot of Paddington, into the bargain – that would otherwise have remained totally unexplored. It was not, I must now shamefacedly admit, entirely unknown for the occasional student to find himself unaccountably lost in one of the now sadly extinct sex shops just down the road in Praed Street, less than a hundred yards from the medical school entrance – and often long after the tutorial would have been due to finish, poor chap.

'Took a wrong turning a couple of hours ago,' he would mutter sheepishly, 'and I'm still struggling to find my way out.'

Whereas lectures were designed to keep the maximum number of students occupied with the minimum hierarchical input, tutorials – cosy little groups of six to eight students in intimate conversation with a member of the otherwise unoccupied teaching staff – were obviously created purely to give all those tutors something to do in the still, quiet hours of their day. These, of course, would be virtually all of them, namely nine to five most Mondays to Fridays, although we must give them some credit for their annual commitment to an introductory lecture at the start of each academic year.

We were also lucky enough to be blessed with personal tutors, an intrinsic component of both our professional development and our unquenchable need to fulfil the 'inner being', which by my definition was the one that had nowhere to go between the hours of closing and reopening in the local public houses. Here was a body of responsible, reliable and trustworthy men and women we could safely approach in times of need . . . difficulty adjusting to the stresses and strains of life away from home, for example; trouble coping with the long hours of work; personal relationships going awry and no one to turn to; inability in the early hours to remember where one lived . . .

My own tutor, George, was a lovely Scotsman – yes, I know this would appear to be a classic example of an oxymoron – with a look of permanent resignation on his face. For some strange reason I could not then comprehend, this seemed to heighten perceptibly whenever I went to see him.

'Lend us a fiver, George,' was a common request upon our meeting.

'Look, Mike,' he would say in exasperation, 'proper students have proper tutorials in their tutors' rooms, sitting on their sofas with cups of herbal tea and the odd joss stick, pouring their hearts out with an occasional sob or two, discussing politics, literature, the meaning of life . . .'

'So that's what proper students do,' I'd muse.

'It's your job to make your tutor feel mature, experienced, valued . . .' he would continue. 'Wanted . . . important . . .'

'But I do value you, George,' I would say in my most reassuring manner, 'I really do. You are important to me. It's not my fault we only ever seem to meet in the pub. Now, about that fiver . . ?'

The end of the seventies and the beginning of the eighties brought the early warning signs that medicine, and medical schools, were about to change for ever. Out of the woodwork and into the lecture theatres slowly, inexorably, like rats rushing into a newly opened sewer, came the happy-clappy, touchy-feely, 'let's go hug a tree' brigade.

No longer, it transpired, were we to say to the patients, 'Tell me, I'm a doctor.' Now we had to empathize, and to share. 'Oh, I spent two weeks with a social worker in Clapham, and the pain, the suffering I saw. Let us together talk through how this most humbling of experiences has changed the way that I view the world, and explore with me the inner demons we both can exorcize, to the fulfilment of us all.'

'Have you got some chicken entrails and a sacrificial virgin?' I always wanted to ask. 'Because I'll be bringing the goat's testicles.'

But not everyone was entirely happy with this shift in emphasis. As Stuart, one of our gynaecological registrars, put it in his typically self-deprecating way, 'I'm very proud of my pedestal, thank you very much, and all I want to do is stay up here for as long as possible. If,' he added drily, 'that's OK with everyone else.'

Stuart's previous claim to fame, if he is to be believed, was that he once owned a nightclub in Liverpool and was approached by the Beatles shortly before they became famous.

'They asked if they could play in the club on a regular basis,' he admitted, adding with a wry smile, 'I gave them a short audition and told them that in my opinion they would never make it in the entertainment business and, in any case, I was putting my faith in Bobby and the Caterpillars instead, so would they please stop bothering me . . . which unfortunately they did.'

Stuart had a nice line in student management.

Generally speaking, clinical teaching – in other words teaching on the wards, with real patients making real grunting and groaning noises somewhere vaguely within touching distance – relied upon that old favourite, trial by ritual student humiliation. This depended heavily upon the fact that the doctor was supposed to know all the answers, while the students generally had little or no idea what they were talking about. Lots of fun would then be had by all concerned in the time it took the former to establish the latter's complete lack of knowledge.

So there we were, in gynaecology outpatients, ten students and Stuart clucking like a mother hen with her most wayward chicks, his gentle words of encouragement ringing in our ears.

'No, not that one, Jenkins,' he would say, with just the right amount of long suffering in his voice.

'S-sorry,' stuttered Jenkins. 'G-glasses got s-steamed up.'

We were all in the process of examining a very pleasant and accommodating lady who had a lump in her abdomen that was so enormous even I had a pretty good notion it should not necessarily have been there.

'Now then, my children,' said Stuart, who for some reason I can no longer recall was universally known as Bilbo (Baggins), 'help me along here. I am a poor struggling registrar who has to go back to my consultant and report upon this delightful lady. Who would like to chip in with a potential diagnosis?'

For once I had made a tactical error on a ward round. Instead of my usual ploy of loitering behind the closed curtains of the bed next door I unaccountably found myself standing immediately to his left, too late for a strategic withdrawal.

'Ah, young Sparrow,' he said genially, spying me before I could escape. 'Ready for one of your usual wild stabs in the dark?'

'Always ready for one of those,' I answered, stroking my chin thoughtfully – a sure sign that, even if I had actually been listening, I had not the faintest idea what the answer was. 'Not pregnant, is she?'

Bilbo turned expressionlessly to the patient. 'How old are you, Mrs Armitage?'

'Seventy-six, dear,' she responded promptly, 'and still got most of my own teeth.'

Bilbo turned back to look at me, totally deadpan. 'Probably not pregnant then,' he agreed, 'and I suppose seeing as how we are in a gynaecology outpatient clinic, and not on the maternity ward, it should have been a bit of a give-away, shouldn't it?'

I nodded humbly. 'If only I had your experience,' I said meekly.

'Right then,' continued Bilbo brightly, after shuddering with mock – at least, I thought it was mock – contempt, 'your best time-wasting manoeuvre now being over, let's have a go at the real answer, shall we? If you know what a real answer actually is.'

15

'Not much point saying ascites?' I ventured. (This is a fluid-like swelling of the stomach, mostly secondary to severe liver disease.)

'Not much,' he agreed, regarding me carefully. 'Tell me, Mike – do you fish?'

'What – I mean, I beg your pardon?' I asked, mystified.

Bilbo grinned. 'It's not a gynaecological question,' he said, 'so there's an outside chance you might come up with the correct answer. Do you fish?'

'No,' I replied confidently, glad that I was going to get at least something right.

'Well, using your imagination – and judging from the answers you normally give to my questions, I know you've got one of those – pretend, if you will, I am out fishing and you are the maggot I have just impaled upon my hook. I would now like you to wriggle a bit.'

'Wriggle?' I said doubtfully.

'Wriggle,' he confirmed, with just the merest hint of a twinkle in his eye, 'whilst I talk to Jenkins, who doesn't need quite such a vivid imagination as you because he has something very useful to offer in the profession you are about to enter. We in the trade refer to it as knowledge.'

So I wriggled dutifully while he spoke to Jenkins, a small, skinny red-haired chap with freckles who probably still had muddy knees beneath his trousers. His poor grasp of topographical anatomy was completely outweighed by his uncanny ability to recite lists of anything you cared to name – shopping, the names of all 101 dalmatians and the order of their birth, and, more pertinently, twenty-one gynaecological causes of gross swelling of the stomach, which was three more than most of the textbooks gave.

'I think it is most likely a cyst,' he began earnestly, a bead of sweat forming on his top lip in his excitement. 'There are fifteen different types of cyst, and I'll give them to you first in

16

alphabetical order, and secondly according to the frequency of their occurrence.'

'Oh no you won't,' said Bilbo hurriedly, glancing across to check I was still wriggling away. 'But Mike, you can try if you like,' he invited, smiling at me so wolfishly that I wondered where I had left my riding hood, and if it was little and red.

Try as I might – and I was well practised at this – I could think of no way out. 'This will come as a bit of a shock to you,' I began, 'but actually – I can't.'

Bilbo raised an eyebrow in mock surprise. 'Really?' he murmured.

'I seem to be lacking in some of the necessary facts,' I explained, acknowledging that continuing to lie was now completely out of the question.

Bilbo stood back in mock consternation.

'Gather ye round, boys and girls – excuse us, Mrs Armitage, this is student-humbling time here, a chance for us all to relax and enjoy the moment – and let us reflect upon a modern miracle. How did this woefully lacking specimen of humanity get so far, knowing so little?'

'Bribery?' suggested Carpenter, a large, rugby-playing Northerner to my left. 'Nepotism, blackmail, impersonating a real student who has been held captive by the Tamil Liberation Army for the past three year?'

'Maybe nobody noticed,' put in Hilary, a slim, quiet girl who rarely spoke unprompted. 'Perhaps he just slipped through by mistake.'

'Enough, enough,' interrupted Bilbo. 'Student baiting is my job – I'm a professional, with years of training to my credit. Let me have another go. Now, has anyone got a piece of paper?'

Strangely enough, Jenkins had. 'A3, A4 or A5?' he asked. 'L-lined, unlined, ch-ch-cheap, middle of the road, or r-r-r-really expensive?'

'Nearest,' said Bilbo, taking the piece offered to him, which he proceeded to fold meticulously in half, and then half again, and kept on folding until he had a wodge the size of a postage stamp.

'Scissors?' he asked, beginning to unfold again, and the outpatient sister duly obliged in the manner of one who, had she been asked for a sabre-toothed tiger with a headache, would have rummaged in her pocket and come up with a phone number where one could have easily been obtained. He cut out a small section of the paper (one sixty-fourth of the original, if you're interested), handed it to me and said, 'There, write down on this every last thing you know about gynaecology. And if you run out of paper, you can turn it over and use the other side.'

Later, when outpatients was over and we were all leaving, Bilbo called me back.

'Sit down for a moment, Mike,' he said. 'All joking over, for now. I want to talk to you.'

I sat as requested, feeling suddenly rather young and vulnerable.

'Look at you, Mike,' he said. 'Despite all the evidence to the contrary I think you're a lovely chap – bright, intelligent, funny, so many things going for you and yet . . .' he shrugged sadly, '. . . and yet you're going nowhere. You seem so absolutely determined just to chuck it all away.'

I opened my mouth to protest, and then closed it again.

'How many people would have given their right arm to be where you are now,' he continued, 'but didn't make it? I could say that you owe it to all those people who would have so loved to be here, but are not, to make a hell of a sight better job of it than you are doing right now. But I'm not going to.'

He sighed and leaned forward, pressing his palms down on the table.

'If you want to be a drifter all your life and end up on the intellectual scrap heap, then just carry on as you are – you're doing it so well as it is you don't need any help from anyone else. But if you actually want to be a doctor, now you've made it through the first couple of years – much to everyone's surprise, I have to say – then for God's sake take a bit of advice. Do a bit of growing up, and do it fast, before it's too late. Try learning a few facts, maybe, revolutionary thought though it might be to you, and why not attend a few lectures, like everybody else? What is it you want – notoriety and a prominent place in the medical school hall of heroic failures, or a degree you can one day do something with and look back on with pride? '

I left, suitably subdued, and wandered off down to Hyde Park for a long walk, and a think.

'Look at me,' he had said as I was leaving. 'I'm you, twenty years from now. I'm forty-three, still a senior registrar, and I should have been here a dozen years ago. If I don't get my consultancy in the next six months I shall probably just have to give up and move on to something else. Is that what you want for yourself?'

He smiled self-deprecatingly, and shrugged again. 'First rule of medicine – never make the same mistake twice. And then there's the second rule – try not to make it in the first place, if you can learn from somebody else who already has. Take a lesson from me, Mike. You can do so much better than this – but only if you want to. All around this hospital there are people who are just dying to see you fail. Prove them wrong – prove them wrong for me, but mostly for yourself.'

I have no idea what became of Bilbo, or where he is now – probably running a bare knuckle boxing booth in the East End, or some such thing – but he taught me some long overdue home truths, for which I belatedly give him my thanks.

Underachiever or not, he was just the type of man that medicine needed then, and needs now even more than ever in these woefully politically correct times.

The undoubted king of the tutorial set, however, was Duncan.

Oh, how can one describe Duncan?

A Donald Sutherland lookalike in his hippy lecturer guise, with brown corduroy jackets, suede shoes and wide knitted ties, he was earnestly shallow, or shallowly earnest, dependent upon your point of view. Most heinously, he taught psychology, and even worse than that, he wrote books about it.

He was obviously a Nicholas Parsons fan.

Nicholas Parsons, for those of you unacquainted with him, was the splendidly urbane presenter of *Sale of the Century*, an ITV quiz programme of the late seventies. Three contestants answered simple general knowledge questions – 'Complete this well-known phrase: Bill and Ben, the Flowerpot . . .' for example – and won the grand sum of £5 for each correct answer. At the end of the programme, the one who had accumulated the most money got to spend it on an array of scintillating prizes – an unassembled MFI wardrobe, a weekend at Pontin's, an ever-popular fondue set – at knockdown prices.

Nicholas would look at the amount of money the winner had to spend, together with the nominal cost of the glorious array of offerings no home should be without, and after various calculations with the aid of a slide rule and a bank of computers he would say, 'Geoffrey, you have already won a waffle maker, a set of stainless steel cutlery and a trip to see Little and Large at Brighton Pavilion . . .' (large round of applause) '. . . and you *still* have £110 left to spend on The Sale of the Century.' (Another round of applause, even louder than before.) 'And I've worked out . . .'

And that was Duncan the tutorial leader, and his first catchphrase.

'And I've worked out . . .' he was always saying, and he didn't mean in the gym, either – one look at a dumbbell and I'm sure he would have felt a migraine coming on.

'And I've worked out,' he said suddenly towards the end of our first session together, leaning forward in his chair to bestow upon us his most earnest 'I am a caring psychologist' look, 'that some of you are not entirely comfortable with yourselves.'

Pretty deep stuff, eh?

Duncan preached free love, at which point the cynics amongst us immediately assumed that he hadn't yet had any and was hoping somebody somewhere would take pity on him and duly oblige. He thought that taking drugs might be trendy, but was careful of inviting ridicule from a group of people normally too inebriated to even care what drugs might be around, let alone make any sort of effort to go and find them. In his more daring moments he would explain that he had once been to a party where he heard that someone was smoking pot in one of the bedrooms, then wait to see our reaction.

He had one other psychological catchphrase – although two in the same psychologist might seem a little too much to bear – which he brought out on a regular basis.

'Ah, Jonathan . . .' he would say earnestly (he never referred to us by our surnames, or nicknames – 'It makes us more of a family,' was his constant explanation, 'and you must call me Duncan'), '. . . late again, keeping the rest of us waiting. How do you feel about that?'

There was a variant on the theme. After, say, a soccer international the evening before, a stirring English win or more realistically another calamitous defeat, he would begin proceedings by writing the result on the blackboard and turning to us to say, 'How do we all *feel* about that?' Or by way of further variation, on occasion, 'How do we all feel about *that?*'

On a good day this might be followed by something like, 'Let us share our thoughts, our feelings, our aspirations, that we might grow together in the complex understanding of each other's relative places in this gloriously unpredictable, this isolationist but ultimately compassionate world of ours, and how we mutually interreact in times of crisis and adversity.'

It was, of course, complete, utter claptrap.

All we ever went for was the potential entertainment value and the need to be registered as having attended a certain percentage of the overall number of tutorials. That, and the hope of all concerned that sooner or later justice would be done and Duncan would fall irrevocably flat on his face.

And, to be honest, none of us wanted to miss the moment.

Because, finally, there was Duncan the role-playing leader. I absolutely loathe role playing at the best of times, but with Duncan . . . I started missing tutorials, much to his relief. He liked to cast himself as some latterday icon and invite us to express our admiration for him – in a purely role-playing capacity, of course.

'It's to help you get in touch with your feelings in a safe, secure environment,' he would ooze nauseously.

And yes, there is a word for this type of man, and no doubt you can think of it just as easily as I.

I suppose it had to happen, sooner or later, but it still came as something of a shock when it finally did.

Rumour had it – a rumour quite possibly circulated by Duncan himself – that he had had a succession of minor affairs with various students over the years. To be honest none of us cared one tenth of an iota, even if we had believed it. After all, if they were to be led astray by Duncan, for goodness sake, then surely they must deserve everything they got.

But all that changed suddenly one day, when Sarah, one of the girls in our year, and our tutorial group, fell unaccountably under his spell. Even that might not have mattered, I suspect, had she not been bright, intelligent, vivacious and unexpectedly pretty, the medical school having obviously committed a crime of unpardonable dimensions by admitting her in the first place.

Most of all, apart from being totally desirable, she was a friend of mine, and I felt partially responsible for not having seen it all coming. Not only that, she came with a ready-made boyfriend back at home by the name of Robert, to whom she had remained disgustingly faithful throughout the entirety of our time at medical school to date, much to the collective disappointment of all my male friends and acquaintances.

As her friends and self-appointed moral guardians – in other words, interfering busybodies – we felt compelled to intervene when we discovered she was becoming rather too friendly with Duncan. I don't as yet have a seventeen-year-old daughter – currently twelve and waiting – but when she gets there I shall already know the best lines.

'But Sarah, he's just too old for you,' I said one day.

'You're so short-sighted,' she said stubbornly, setting her jaw with that 'Whatever you say isn't going to make any difference' look that I knew so well. 'And so juvenile. Age no longer matters in these enlightened times – I can *talk* to him, really talk, and he's interested in me as a *person*.'

Yeah right, I thought cynically, being for once wise enough not to put it into words.

'But you can talk to me,' I countered, trying to sound deeply upset and wounded and, if I may say so myself, making rather a good job of it, too.

'But that's completely different,' she said irritatedly, shaking her head in frustration. 'No, I can't explain, but he's just so . . . mature, so grown up and you're just . . . well, Mike, maturity isn't the first word any of us would use to describe you, is it?'

Now that hurt, though I like to think I rose above it with dignity.

I even tried, 'But he's so shallow, it must be obvious he's only interested in one thing,' only to have it reflected back as, 'He's got hidden depths. Trust *you* not to see them.'

But I knew it was truly serious when in a fit of desperation one day I said, 'For goodness sake, Sarah, he's got sideburns!' followed shortly afterwards by a judiciously murmured, 'And what would Robert think?' This, sadly, resulted in an even firmer set of the jaw, an end to the conversation and a refusal to talk to me for the rest of the week.

Matters had to come to a head sooner or later, and duly they did.

Arriving back from a party in the early hours one morning with Neil – my flatmate – and Kim, Sarah's closest friend, we spied Duncan sliding out of the front door of the medical school hall of residence whistling tunelessly, a self-satisfied grin on his face.

'Uh-oh,' I murmured, 'I'm not sure I like the look of this . . .'

The next day, as I remained distinctly *persona non grata*, Kim approached her tentatively.

'Sarah,' she said, 'Mike, Neil and I were coming back here late last night and we saw Duncan leaving with a silly grin on his face. Sarah, you didn't, did you? What on earth do you think you are doing? What about Robert?'

'It's none of your business and it's none of *his* business,' she exploded forcefully, 'so why don't the pair of you just leave me alone? And no, I didn't,' she added, 'but I bloody well will if I want to!'

Something had to be done, and soon. That much was obvious. It was just the what, the when and the where that were proving a bit difficult to figure out.

A week later I was returning from the pub with Neil, Kim and Sarah after a hatchet-burying session. Sarah, we had all agreed, must be allowed to make her own choices in life – even if we totally disagreed with them – and we apologized profusely for sticking our noses into what was obviously her private affair. We were just worried about her, we had explained, and had taken our concern too far, albeit in what we felt to be her best interests.

We had solemnly promised to leave her completely alone from that point onwards, to make her own decisions and her own mistakes, if so they proved to be. Our apologies were duly accepted, and peace at last reigned, for the time being.

Or at least, it did until we neared Wilson House, the medical school hall of residence, where there was a bit of a commotion going on.

A man who appeared at first sight to be only partially dressed, and at second sight not dressed at all, was banging on the side door at the end of the crescent in front of the building where the residents parked their cars.

'Let me in,' a voice hissed urgently, 'for God's sake let me in before somebody recognizes me. I've got no clothes on.'

I felt Sarah stiffen imperceptibly beside me. As we drew nearer a first-floor sash window flew violently open, and a woman, naked from the waist upwards, with her arms folded discreetly across her chest, leaned out and called down, 'First time I go out with a psychologist, and just my luck to get an impotent one. You are a sad and pathetic man, Duncan Jefferson, and I wish I had listened to my friends.'

She disappeared just as suddenly from view, and the window snapped shut again.

Duncan, his back to the door, slid abjectly down to the ground, one hand covering his eyes, the other his so recently denigrated manhood.

'Let me in,' he called again feebly. 'This is all just a bad dream.'

We were now only a couple of yards away, and Sarah was staring open-mouthed at the spectacle before her. Her eyes met Duncan's, and he scrambled to his feet, appalled.

'I can explain,' he said desperately. 'I can explain . . .'

'Now that would be interesting to hear,' whispered Kim in my ear.

But whatever the explanation might have been we never got around to hearing it, for at precisely that moment a taxi screeched round the corner and drew to a halt in front of us. A well-dressed, long-legged blonde stepped elegantly out, walked three paces forward and stood, hands on her hips, looking in total disdain at our somewhat disadvantaged psychologist.

'So everything they said about you was true,' she said with contempt. 'Well, needless to say, Mr Duncan bloody Jefferson, the engagement's off, and I never, ever, want to see you again in my entire life.'

And with that she wrenched an engagement ring from her finger, hurled it venomously at him, stepped just as elegantly back into the taxi and was gone before any of us had a chance to draw breath.

I felt a small tug on my arm. It was Sarah.

'Take me away from here, Mike, please,' she said in a small voice. 'Anywhere. Just take me away.'

A month later Sarah was back to her old self, and Duncan a hollow shell of a man.

I was sitting one morning having a cup of coffee with Kim in the medical school refectory.

'Nice to see Sarah back to normal,' she said casually.

'Yes, nice,' I agreed absently.

'Strange how all that should happen when we were out at the pub together,' continued Kim, looking at me pointedly.

'Yes, strange,' I agreed, as if I had something else of burning importance on my mind.

'And isn't it odd how nobody else knew that Duncan was already engaged?' she persisted.

'Not really,' I said, hesitating. 'In fact, if you must know, Duncan hadn't actually realized he was engaged himself . . .'

It had taken a bit of organization, but nothing beyond our limited capabilities. The unexpected 'fiancée' was Neil's sister, just returned from three years in Australia and unknown to all, and the girl in the upstairs room in Wilson House was Cherice, Neil's sister's friend, a woman of great spirit and enterprise whose acquaintance I was keen to pursue further.

We had borrowed a room — sort of without the occupant's knowledge as they were away on holiday at the time, my just happening to have the pass keys in my possession — and she had enticed Duncan back after a 'chance' meeting in the pub, each with a slightly different agenda in mind.

The rest, as they say, was history.

I have only one regret.

As I had led Sarah away from Wilson House the side door flew suddenly open and in tumbled the less than fully attired Duncan, landing flat on his back on the floor. Looking up in horror he found himself amidst the fully assembled remainder of our tutorial group, together with a carefully invited handful of one or two friends and interested bystanders.

And I missed it.

'Well, Duncan,' said the wonderful Cherice, now fully clothed once more, 'here you lie cowering, naked and alone, and then not quite so alone after all. Your reputation and your lack of endowment stand fully exposed for each and every one of us to see, and yet what we want to know is – all together everybody – what we really want to know is . . .'

'So how do you feel about that?' chorused one and all.

2

Anything for a Bet

'Whatever you do,' Oscar had said, 'do it with confidence.'

Well, we tried, we really did. It's just that confidence stems from knowledge of one's subject, experience in the relevant disease processes, and an innate understanding of the patient's condition . . . and we didn't have any.

But it wasn't our fault.

These days students are exposed to real patients (or is it the other way round?) early in their careers, but this was back in the dark ages of the late 1970s when the height of our expectation was to insert the thermometer in the correct orifice after no more than three attempts, and occasionally the right way round. Our first two years of incredibly exciting study were spent in a series of gloomy lecture theatres long before we ever encountered a real patient. During these first revelatory six terms we learned, for example, everything you could ever wish to know about biochemistry, and then a little bit more.

'See, it can be fun,' said our lecturer, adding one clear liquid to another and watching a single small bubble emerge from the colourless mixture over a week later. How lucky he was to be able to travel through life so easily sustained by such simple pleasures. And if it wasn't biochemistry on our delectable menu then – oh joy – it was physiology, pharmacology or anatomy. Can you imagine how thrilling it can be to dissect an armpit?

At the start of our third year the great day of our inaugural visit to the wards finally arrived, and along with that came 'The Big Moment'. It was like some sort of inverse initiation ceremony. In West Africa young tribesmen are sent out to go and kill their first lion bare-handed, with only the aid of their loin-cloth; nomads in Outer Mongolia are circumcised without recourse to a local anaesthetic; in the Great Outback aborigines celebrate when their first boomerang comes back sometime the same day they threw it. But in Paddington . . .

For two years we had been striding fearlessly down the medical school corridors in the long white coat of the dissection room – well, it had a passing resemblance to being white when we started, but somehow always managed to transform into a sort of bodily fluid-stained yellowy grey by the middle of the second week. The smell of the sluice room beckoned. Our moment was nigh.

Echoing the haunting shriek of the novice vampire drawing blood from his first unsuspecting victim as he sinks his newly grown fangs into their fatally exposed neck, we emerged triumphantly from the laundry room bearing our long-awaited prize . . .

The short, trendy white coat, all the better to swagger around hospital corridors in.

And why, I hear you ask, did we need a short white coat in the first place? Was it because we were obliged to hack the bottom off the original article with a pair of pinking shears to shed all the evidence of that blood and formalin which might otherwise have spattered over our trousers? No, most definitely not – the sole underlying reason was to distinguish us from that eminently superior breed, the real doctors, the qualified ones, who were back in their long white coats again. Confusing, isn't it?

It was, as we later learned and came to fully support, of the utmost importance for all concerned to be able instantly to differentiate the students from their elders and – as I now understand myself to be – substantially betters. For a start, it allowed the already severely put-upon patients on the wards to inform us firmly and with intent, 'No, you may not insert your index finger into my rectum for purely educational purposes,' but there was a far more crucial significance than that.

It greatly assisted the student nurses to recognize – and consequently avoid – us at mess parties.

Late September, 1977. I remember it well.

There we were, sitting in our first outpatients session full of hope, apprehension and a whole array of minor tranquillizers. Behind his desk sat our overlord, Mr Broadbent, the consultant surgeon, surveying the scene with a thoughtful expression, and before him an array of eight students, all of us feeling unaccustomedly nervous and out of place, like the new boy in the grammar school wearing short trousers when the recognized dress was long.

He was patently obviously in the wrong job. You could tell at a glance. A kindly, avuncular chap with grey hair receding to his spinal column, he should have been running a neighbourhood sweet shop in a quaint Olde Worlde village somewhere in Middle England, bestowing gob-stoppers and aniseed balls upon his best customers' young children, instead of injecting pulsatile haemorrhoids and piercing subterranean cysts with a 'Could be something innocent' smile upon his face.

'Right, gentlemen,' he began, smiling disarmingly – there being no women amongst us, probably to their great relief. 'We will today be presented with something in excess of twenty patients with a variety of surgical problems, ranging from the deadly serious to the totally insignificant. A percentage of them will have been sent along by their GPs for a first appointment, and will be nervous, or truculent, or both. Some will be back for review, having been exposed to our tender mercies on at least one previous occasion, and one or two may have come directly from casualty for an urgent opinion. Everyone with me so far?'

We all nodded vigorously, too overawed to speak.

'A rowdy lot, aren't you?' he observed with a good-humoured

frown. 'To continue, then. You have to bear in mind that probably one in every five of them will find something to complain about, if you but give them the opportunity. The best advice I can offer you, should this happen, is to insist they completely disrobe behind the cubicle curtain in order that you are able to give them the comprehensive examination they so obviously deserve. This will also allow you to hide a critical article of their clothing when their back is turned.' He winked solemnly at us. 'They won't be complaining for long.'

We all chuckled nervously.

Much to our collective surprise Mr Broadbent seemed disconcertingly normal, a fully paid-up member of the human race, and we hadn't been adequately prepared for this. No doubt it would quickly pass, I reassured myself. Given time he would surely metamorphose into a sinister version of Darth Vader's elder brother, or grow two little horns from his temples and dribble green slime out of the corner of his mouth, just like all the rest of them.

'Right then,' he continued, a look of wry amusement on his face. 'I assume you've all been taught the basic rules of examining patients, haven't you?'

Again we all nodded, each waiting for somebody else to break the silence.

'Goodness, you're a quiet bunch,' he said, smiling broadly. 'OK, can anyone tell me what the first step in the comprehensive assessment of our patient should be?'

It wasn't supposed to happen.

None of us there could have anticipated it, most especially me, but I just couldn't help it – it came out in an unexpected rush before I could stop myself. I gave him the right answer.

'Take a history, sir,' I said.

'Very good, young man,' he said, duly impressed. 'And you are?'

'A little nervous,' I admitted.

31

'I was thinking more in terms of your name,' he replied, biting his lip.

'Oh, Sparrow, sir,' I answered, blushing a dusky shade of vermilion.

'Indeed.' He lowered his glasses and regarded me over them with those benign, intelligent eyes. 'Are you sure?'

'About taking a history?' I closed my eyes briefly, and took a deep breath. 'Yes, sir, I think so.'

'No, that's not what I meant,' he said, stifling a snort.

You could tell he wanted to laugh, but was just managing to rein himself in. 'Are you sure about being Sparrow?' he continued with impressive self-control. 'You're not some sort of impostor, are you, out to make a name for himself? From what they told me I would have expected a response more along the lines of "Don't touch the patient until you are satisfied he's not actively contagious," or "Pretend the fire alarm's gone off and rush into casualty looking for something to extinguish."'

'He's not feeling himself today, sir,' said the chap sitting next to me. 'Please try not to worry – it's a bit like the BBC during a concerted spell of atmospheric interference. Normal service will be resumed by the end of the week.'

Mr Broadbent turned his mild-mannered glance to my immediate neighbour.

'So if he's Sparrow,' he said slowly, perusing the list of names in front of him, 'then you must be . . . '

'Callaghan, sir.'

'Ah yes, Callaghan.' He looked up, a mixture of emotions on his face. '"Skid" Callaghan, it apparently says down here, although to what the "Skid" relates appears to have been – fortunately for us all – obliterated by something unmentionable one of the outpatient nurses has spilt over my checklist. Yes,' he admitted shrewdly, 'they warned me about you as well. Several times, in fact – and some of them in writing.'

But still he said it with that gentle smile on his face, the mark of a true gentleman – or a man who knows no fear, and possibly no reason.

'But I said I would teach the pair of you, anyway,' he added drolly. 'If that's all right with you both?'

'Oh yes, sir, fine, sir. Certainly, sir,' we agreed hastily, all the while wondering when the men in the white coats with their strait-jackets were going to come and take him away.

'Splendid,' murmured Mr Broadbent, and 'Splendid,' he repeated again, a little more doubtfully this time. 'Now, let us see what we can find for you to do today.'

He had just begun to study the pile of notes in front of him when the door to his left swung open, and in came the sister in charge of outpatients with a mesmeric sway of her hips.

'Ah, Julia,' he said, smiling beatifically. 'A great pleasure to see you, as always. I'm looking for a suitable case for Sparrow and Callaghan to take on – that is those two young rascals on the end there. Perhaps you already know them?'

'Oh, I do, sir,' she said, wrinkling her nose deliciously. 'We all know Sparrow and Callaghan here, sir.' She leaned across his desk and selected a set of notes from the available choices for all the world as if she was picking the ripest plum from the best tree in the orchard.

'This, sir, as I am sure you will agree, will almost certainly be the making of them.'

Mr Broadbent flicked over a couple of pages, and tried unsuccessfully to suppress a snort.

'Just the thing,' he agreed, temporarily unable to meet our eyes. 'So, off you go, gentlemen – you'll be wanting cubicle number two, through the door behind you and down on your left. Back here to report to us all in fifteen minutes at the most, if you please.'

Now, like the majority of people when I arrived at medical school, I like to think I was fairly prejudice free. I didn't mind black or white or yellow; smokers or anti-smokers; fat, thin, clean or smelly – no, that's a lie, I seriously minded fat and smelly – but in all other respects I was prepared to treat almost anyone, no matter how unsavoury their person, their disease or their political affiliations.

But five years of the most intense indoctrination at medical school changed all that, altering my perceptions beyond all I had previously held to be credible. I emerged in due course triumphant, proudly waving my hard-earned certificate of unmitigated bias along with the best of them.

Our bias – even in those days – was scrupulously politically correct, in line with the best of modern-day philosophies. We treated everybody as equals – which to our way of thinking meant being equally prejudiced against the lot of them. But although we hated all patients, whatever their disease, body odour or site of purulent discharge, irrespective of their colour, creed or football club loyalties, our particular contempt was reserved for the chosen few.

The Welsh, of course, were inevitably at the top of any list – too good at rugby (I am talking about a quarter of a century ago) and too unbearable in a crowd of more than two. They were invariably closely followed by the Americans – too much money, too little dress sense and too corpulent to be accorded any form of respect. Yes, I know this is a sweeping generalization, but it is more fun that way. The third runner-up, to borrow a phrase from that now archaic institution, Miss World, was anyone who spoke in a language we didn't understand, which included most Brummies and every Liverpudlian we had ever met.

It is just possible some of them may have quite unreasonably had a less than favourable opinion of ourselves, but did we care?

There was, however, one central tenet to the institutional dyspepticism in which we were all united – we abhorred the Australians. A favourite joke of the time – well, amongst the English – was as follows: What's the difference between Australia and a yoghurt? Given time, even yoghurt will develop a culture.

As an ageing GP I am now of course devoid of such irrational dislikes, but at the time Skid Callaghan and I left the office for cubicle number two I had just become a fully paid-up member of the National Xenophobic Society, shortly to be running for president. But all that was to change in the blink of an eye . . .

As we tentatively opened the cubicle door and stepped inside, our jaws fell to the ground. I have often since believed that when it came to picking them up again I must have inadvertently acquired the other bit of Skid's by mistake, as it has never appeared to fit quite as snugly since.

For there she stood before us, an Australian goddess. All those hours, all those days we had spent swapping sheep-shearing and Rolf Harris jokes, all those nights we had tried to pretend that *Mad Max II* wasn't the best film that has ever been made, all the sweatshop labour we had put into building up and reinforcing our Antipodean prejudices just evaporated, in an instant, never to return.

She was tall, tanned, with flowing golden hair and a figure to die for. There were six knees in that small room, and I knew for a fact that at least four of them were trembling.

She cocked an eyebrow at us and smiled broadly.

'Hello, boys,' she drawled seductively, and I was immediately struck with amazement that I could have ever thought the Australian accent even vaguely unattractive. 'Have you come to sort me out?'

There was just one thought uppermost in my mind. Whatever it is that might be wrong with her, I prayed silently, please don't let it be something she has to take any of her clothes off for.

It's a strange paradox in medicine, this, one widely known as the Law of Inverse Disrobing. Medicine is one of the few professions – I challenge you to think of another – where people regularly take their clothes off in front of you without any money changing hands. The more you would like a member of the appropriate sex to take their clothes off in front of you should you be alone together somewhere private once the pubs have closed, and the greater the size of their expense account with Janet Reger, the less you can cope with the equivalent event in your surgery.

Old ladies with twelve layers of underwear in mid-July who want you to inspect their umbilical hernia during the busiest surgery of the decade – no problem. Elderly gentlemen the size of whose prostates just begs to be assessed due to their equal inability to urinate less than three times an hour and to remove their braces and whalebone corsets in less than half an hour – it's just a pleasure. But give me a quiet afternoon, an absence of paperwork (dream on) and a gorgeous female patient with only the sheerest of silk next to her delicately tanned skin who has a rash she just must show me before it fades away, and I start mumbling, 'No, no, I think I know what it is . . . '

'But you haven't seen it,' she complains. 'Don't you just want to take a look?'

'I'm learning to be psychic,' I lie feebly. 'It's a new concept known as diagnosis by thought transference.'

'You can see it best if I take my top off.'

'Do you not have a bit somewhere below the wrist I can have a peek at?' I counter desperately.

'No, I don't,' she replies firmly, undoing the zip on her skirt, ' and the best of it is here, just at the top of my leg.'

There's only one way out of this that I know, and it seems to work pretty much every time.

'I think I need a second opinion,' I mumble. 'My receptionist lives only a couple of doors down from a consultant dermatologist. I'll ask her to take a look . . . '

Back to Ellie, as our goddess turned out to be called, who stood, hand on delectably jutting out hip and a tantalizing smile curling the corners of a pair of lips that could have peeled a lemon without breaking sweat.

Skid Callaghan and I looked at each other, swallowed hard and moved uneasily into our respective well-rehearsed history-taking techniques.

'Um . . . ' I began, before lapsing into silence.

'Well . . . ' started Skid, as if he was convinced he at least knew what he was going to say next, but was not quite so certain when he was going to start saying it. 'Well . . . '

'Um . . . ' I added again helpfully, and then suddenly we all got a fit of the giggles, except that we giggled like schoolboys while she . . . she giggled beautifully. There was only one way to regain the last vestiges of our dignity.

'Well, John,' I said slowly, 'do you think she's noticed we're a bit nervous?'

'I think she might have,' he said slowly, as Ellie nodded solemnly in front of us, her eyes brimming with laughter.

'So what's exactly wrong with you?' I finally ventured to ask, breaking the short silence following Skid's whispered 'Please be gentle with us. We're new to this. This is our first time.'

'I've got a boil on me bum,' she said with a directness that was almost as disturbing as the diagnosis itself. Almost – but not quite.

Why? I thought desperately. You could have had a boil anywhere – your heel, your elbow, on the end of your nose. Why did it have to be on your bum?

You could have cut the atmosphere with a soggy paper bag, should you have had one to hand.

'Um,' I volunteered eventually, after what seemed like a couple of weeks' delay, 'how long have you had it?'

'All my life,' she said seriously. 'I don't know about you Englishmen, but most of us Australians are born with one.'

For a couple of seconds I thought we had strayed into a Monty Python sketch, and then I realized what she meant. By a series of stumbling steps we haltingly established the size, location and longevity of the offending carbuncle. As dutiful students we then continued to enquire regarding its firmness and degree of pain, following which we discussed the relative merits of surgical intervention as opposed to antibiotic therapy.

'Well, thank you,' I said at last, having run out of questions to ask.

'Yes, thank you,' echoed Skid enthusiastically

'We'll, um . . . ' I began.

' . . . go back to report,' finished Skid. 'To our consultant.'

'Yes, we'll go back to report,' I agreed thankfully, and together we shot out of the cubicle as fast as we could, only narrowly avoiding getting jammed in the doorway.

'So,' said Mr Broadbent as we returned to his room, pale and sweating profusely, 'what have you got to tell me?'

We shuffled our feet nervously in front of him, neither of us all that desperate to speak. He inspected us in his avuncular fashion over the rim of his glasses. 'Come on, gentlemen,' he said, 'you've just seen a patient and we are all bursting to hear what you think of her. Share it with us, do. It hasn't been re-classified as a state secret in your short journey back from cubicle two, has it?'

'Oh, no sir,' we reassured him together. 'It's just that . . . she just . . . we only . . . '

'Did you actually take a look at her pathology?' he asked shrewdly.

We exchanged glances. 'Oh, you wanted us to *look* at it, did you?' I said lamely.

'It's always a help,' he agreed. 'Off you go again, boys. And don't keep us waiting all week.'

'He sent you back to take a look at it, didn't he?' said Ellie, trying unsuccessfully to suppress a smile.

'Yes,' we nodded sheepishly.

The moment we were both dreading had finally arrived. I

tried desperately to think of something, anything that would delay it but before I could do so she unceremoniously un- buttoned her Levis, wriggled her hips deliciously as she slid them down and said, 'Are you ready for this now?'

'No, not at all,' I said immediately, and 'Yes, I rather think I am,' contributed Skid at one and the same time.

So we looked, from a variety of angles and distances. All things considered, I think we got rather a good view, and when it was all over she rebuttoned her Levis as casually as if she were doing up her shoelaces and just stood there, smiling at us. 'Anything else you would like to take a look at, boys?'

'Loads,' we replied in unison, 'but sadly none of it all that medically relevant.'

We dragged ourselves reluctantly back to outpatients again, reported our findings to Mr Broadbent and our envious col- leagues between bouts of uncontrollable shaking, and then went in search of the longest, coldest shower the capital city could provide.

But there is of course more to outpatients than just sick people. There are the doctors, for a start, who are usually greatly more in need of tender loving care than anyone else present, and we mustn't forget the nurses – try as we would sometimes like to.

And as for the patients – well, some of those present (and this may come as a bit of a shock to those of you of a delicate disposition) are no more ill than are you and I. They were just referred in all good faith several years previously, and those who were not actually dead by the time they finally received an appointment have decided to turn up out of sheer curiosity to find out what was originally wrong with them all that time ago.

You meet some very strange people in outpatient waiting rooms. How else can you explain the presence of men at a gynae- cological gathering, unless they fell asleep at the men's health clinic the day before and woke up with such a hell of a shock they were unable to effect an escape? What about adults at a paediatric session? They had probably been referred as a six-year-old but not received an appointment until the painful memories of puberty had long since been forgotten. And who would willingly attend a 'Psychosexual therapy for the completely inadequate in every respect' clinic?

And no, if you are wondering, I am not making it up, it takes place on the third Thursday of each month at a well-known hospital in the Midlands, and I have been there – albeit in a purely observational capacity. I've even tried to refer half a dozen patients there myself over the past few years, there being no local equivalent, but my typist tells me she has been unable to interpret the terminal case of giggles on the Dictaphone.

A constant source of irritation at every outpatient session were the DNAs. Deoxy ribonucleic acid as discovered by Watson and Crick, you may ask? Dangerously Neurotic Adolescents? Or simply Dead and Not Available?

No, the truth was far more mundane and boring, but open to the endless interpretation of idle minds and wandering fingers. They were the Did Not Attends, and what self-respecting student could possibly resist the infinite possibilities thus engendered?

We rarely, as undergraduates, indulged in betting, being too impecunious to risk our hard-earned drinking allowance on such frivolous activities. Neither did we gamble (well, OK, we did a bit) because we could none of us afford to win or lose each other's money, and we most definitely did not sell our bodies into the cause of science – or at least, not more than once. The money was good, but the general discomfiture and resulting side effects were just not worth the recompense, as I discovered to my cost after spending eight hours immobilized in a laboratory chair with three tubes in my stomach and a drip in each arm whilst a slightly wild-eyed professor took regular blood samples to check upon a hormone I had never even heard of. Come to think of it, I still haven't.

The exception to all this, however, was Thomas. Tall, blond and blue-eyed, he paid regular visits to the sperm bank and left with more than just a smile on his face. Sadly for me, there wasn't quite the same market for ginger hair, a big nose and freckles . . .

But boy, could we accept a dare, and pay a forfeit.

'I dare you to turn up to three histology lectures in a row,' ventured my flatmate, knowing full well he was on to a winner.

'I dare you to turn up to a meeting of the black lesbian vegetarian CND society and request associate membership,' I countered politely.

Too easy, of course. 'I bet you couldn't take the place of a DNA and get away with it,' came back the challenge. 'In Mr Frankham's clinic.'

Now *that* was something to think seriously about.

Mr Frankham, let's face it, was an eccentric on a grand scale. In today's politically correct health service he would no doubt have long since been drummed out of the NHS for unadulterated weirdism, and in some far-off century or other he would probably have been burned at the stake. At St Mary's, however, he was a consultant orthopaedic surgeon of some repute, and deemed to be verging on the normal, which is a bit like saying Attila the Hun could be occasionally tetchy.

My children have taken drama lessons from an early age, but until this moment the thespian in me had remained dormant. The nearest I ever got to an equivalent deception was pretending to be interested in neurophysiology for a whole week, not because it was inherently fascinating so much as because the neurophysiologist was on holiday and his stand-in was just so much prettier.

And so the big moment finally came. The bet was on.

There I was, sitting in outpatients, with a card in my hand stating unequivocally that I was one Marcus Jenkins with an internally deranged knee joint. There were only two minor problems to overcome: there was nothing actually wrong with either of my knees, and Marcus was an Afro-Caribbean immigrant, whereas I wasn't.

So I improvised.

Mr Frankham, whom I had in fact never met, was renowned for being originally an inhabitant of an alternative solar system. Rumour had it that his immediate progenitor came from the planet Zog, and being the product of an asexual reproductive process initiating from a small bud somewhere to the south of his mother's left elbow he could smell an impostor a mile distant in a force ten hurricane.

I reluctantly decided, therefore, to dispense with the Black and White Minstrel Show make-up, refused point blank to wear the acrylic wig or have my lips injected with collagen, and emphatically vetoed the once in a lifetime opportunity to have my face and hands blacked with boot polish.

And no, this had nothing to do with institutional racism – it was just too damned uncomfortable.

When we were at the 'I bet you wouldn't do that' stage, it had seemed like a positively splendid idea.

'You don't look very ethnic to me,' said the sister in charge of outpatients dubiously, as I checked in.

'I don't really feel it,' I replied sweetly. 'England is my adopted mother country, and I feel that I belong here, now. I feel quite at home.'

But all the time I was wondering, not for the first time in my life, what exactly I thought I was doing.

I was diverted, however, by the strange behaviour of the chap sitting opposite me. He was busy muttering something malevolent-sounding under his breath – which is not, I have to say, an altogether unusual occurrence in Paddington. It's just that most of the under-the-breath mutterers of my previous acquaintance tended to sleep in gutters clutching empty bottles of meths and milk, or would turn up unannounced at psychiatric outpatients, demanding to be seen.

This guy, intriguingly, was wearing an expensive if slightly grubby overcoat over an immaculate Armani suit, sported an obvious wig and appeared to be sadly in need of a better pair of glasses as he was peering short-sightedly through some tortoise-shell monstrosities at a local newspaper.

He had also – and I noticed this only because I happen to have the same – a deformed left little finger, which like mine must once have been dislocated and failed to be reinstated in precisely the right position. I suspected, however, that he had not sustained this major injury in quite the same fashion as I had, by falling off his nephew's very small bike.

But even more intriguing than that, he had propped up against the wall by the side of his seat a couple of sandwich boards. We all know those people who patrol up and down the London pavements bearing the glad tidings that 'The end of the world is nigh,' or 'Get your suppositories from Superdrug,' but his were rather different. On the side of one I could read the words 'Down with all hospital consultants,' and on another the slightly ominous rhetorical question 'Who wants to wait on a waiting list anyway?'

Ten minutes later, things began to get interesting.

Mr Frankham was late, for a start, and it was now a good three-quarters of an hour after the first patient was due to be seen. There was not a doctor in sight, let alone a consultant, the only action of note being when the sister in charge of outpatients stuck her head around the door every five minutes announcing brightly, 'He won't be long now.'

'And what precisely does that mean?' demanded Sandwich Man menacingly. 'Are we talking this side of Christmas?'

'Oh yes,' came the slightly forced reply. 'Ha, ha, ha. We do so love it here when you patients have your little joke with us.'

'So which Christmas are we talking about,' I asked, throwing what caution I had left to the four winds. 'This one, the next one, or one of the several after that?'

'Ha, ha, ha,' she repeated desperately, and then withdrew behind the safety of the door again, closing it firmly in her wake.

Sandwich Man glanced across at me, and then beckoned with a well-manicured forefinger to the empty seat next to him.

'A word with you, young man,' he said imperiously, adding as I regarded him with more than a little suspicion, 'if you please.'

In for a penny, I thought, wandering curiously across to see what he had in mind.

He put his hand up to his mouth and whispered behind it, 'How would you feel about a little demonstration?'

'Of what?' I whispered back. 'Swedish massage? Flower arranging? How to squeeze twelve people waiting in an out-patient department into the front seat of a Mini?'

'Against the wait,' he said, rightly oblivious to my childish sarcasm. 'Let's teach these hospital consultants a thing or two. It's time we patients showed them we are no longer prepared to accept such shoddy treatment. We should get them to take their responsibilities more seriously. Now is the time to utilize the untapped forces of patient power, draw strength from the groundswell of public opinion, lead the silent majority in a splendid uprising through the streets of London . . . '

'There's only seven of us here,' I reminded him gently.

'Eight,' he corrected adroitly as another rebel-to-be joined our cause. 'And there may be twenty million Manchester United supporters worldwide, but somebody had to be the first one.'

He gathered his placards together, and handed me one. 'Where's your spirit of adventure? Are you with me, or are you for ever going to be suppressed by the enemies of hunting, free speech and obligatory cod liver oil for all our children?'

'No,' I meant to say firmly, 'I'm not with you at all,' but there was something compellingly authoritative about the way he put it that seemed to brook no argument.

'Um, yes,' I found myself saying decisively, reaching out for a placard. 'Yes. Lead on, sir, whoever you may be, and you'll find I'm right behind you.'

'Oh good,' he said, a mischievous look appearing in his eyes. 'Let's give it all we have got.'

He held out his hands in front of him and started slowly to clap.

'Oh, why are we waiting?' he sang in a deep baritone. 'Why-y are we waiting . . .'

'Oh, why are we wai-ai-ting?' somebody joined in enthusiastically, and to my abject horror I realized it was me.

As everyone else began to participate, first timorously and then with the utmost vigour, we rose to our feet as one, and started marching. Round and round the outpatient department we strode, proudly declaring our stated intent, and then we were off, down the nearest corridor towards the urology clinic, bursting triumphantly through a side door into the intensive care unit with our leader magnificent and unbowed at the head of our disparate group, chanting his little heart out. And I followed, dancing and cheering with the best of them as we headed towards the hospital entrance, passers-by stopping and staring in our wake.

It was madness, sheer unadulterated mayhem; it was gloriously, irreverently chaotic. It was magnificent and yet senseless at one and the same time. It was doomed to failure . . .

'Hold this for me for a moment, would you?' said Sandwich Man, passing me a banner he had unfurled from his pocket some two blocks down from the mortuary. 'There's something I have to do.'

'Down with the Professor of Orthopaedic Surgery,' I read out loud, and grinned demonically.

I held it aloft self-importantly, and sang, and danced, and exhorted our ever-enlarging entourage some more . . . until Sandwich Man disappeared suddenly from view in the vicinity of the stool culture collection unit immediately adjacent to the gastro-enterology department and I found myself alone at the head of what seemed like several hundred or more demonstrators, clutching the banner he had so trustingly bequeathed to me as if my very life depended on it.

I looked around, threw what little caution there was left to the wind and set off purposefully down the corridor. They followed me blindly, unfailingly loyal as if they were the rats and the children of Hamlyn and I the Pied Piper.

I felt elated. It was one of those rare yet gloriously momentous occasions suspended for ever in a vacuum of time — I was the spearhead of a new revolution, invincible, indefatigable, focusing the power of the people through the magnifying glass of life on to the smouldering reality of patient dissatisfaction. Now, surely now we could carry the weight of all public opinion before us.

And then I saw the Professor of Surgery heading forcefully down the corridor towards us, just a few seconds before he saw me. My number, I suddenly realized, was very much about to be up.

I took a deep breath, looked frantically around, and swallowing my pride slipped away under the cover of a passing couple of auxiliaries heading for the sluice room with a collection of bedpans. For the next fifteen minutes I cowered behind the door of the ladies' loo until my worthy band of followers had moved on, rudderless, finally to disperse in a state of complete disarray in the barren wastelands between the staff canteen and the prosthetic limb lost property department.

When all appeared to be quiet I sneaked humbly back to outpatients — after all, a bet was a bet — and found I was the only patient there. The sister emerged through the door a few seconds after my arrival and announced brightly, 'Queue's shortened a bit, hasn't it? What have you done with them all? Led them away on a march through the hospital, ha, ha, ha?'

'Yes,' I replied honestly.

'Oh, you are a one,' she responded gleefully. 'Come on then, Marcus. Come through to Doctor.'

I was trapped.

I could just see the headlines. 'Student impersonates Afro-Caribbean (badly) and leads riot in teaching hospital.' 'Career glorious but short-lived.' 'How can one man be so stupid, and so often?'

There are times in your life when you have to take a deep breath, grit your teeth, gird whatever loins you happen to be left with and bite the bullet, going with whatever flow you think you can still hold on to – but this quite obviously wasn't one of them. I stood up to run away, but the sister grabbed hold of me cheerfully and led me through the portals of doom, and to my nemesis.

'Ah, Marcus Jenkins,' said the balding, well-spoken man before me in clipped, Old Etonian tones. 'I am given to understand you lead a life subjugated to the deleterious effects of an internally deranged knee.'

'Um, yes,' I said, surprised that I had lasted this far and wondering what 'deleterious' and 'subjugated' meant. Twenty seconds and counting.

'Which knee is it, exactly?' he asked, narrowing his eyes.

I looked down at my legs, still one on each side. Research is everything, they say, which may explain why I have never made much of a journalist.

'So . . . um . . . which does it say in your notes?' I asked innocently. 'I've had trouble with them both, you see, and you can't rely on anyone to get it absolutely right these days, can you? My GP does his best of course, but . . . '

'Right,' said Mr Frankham deliberately.

'Oh good,' I breathed thankfully, 'because right it is.'

You must all know that moment – the one when in the depths of adversity you have pulled the proverbial rabbit out of the bag; when you have triumphed against unaccountable odds whilst all around you are failing; when you have scaled the heights of Everest when all others remain firmly ensconced in the doldrums. It's a wonderfully exhilarating, life-reinforcing feeling . . . but sadly it wasn't one I was about to have now.

'Left,' he said, pushing the notes towards me, adding pointedly as I stared unblinkingly at the patient details in front of me, 'and you're not in fact an unadulterated Afro-Caribbean, are you?'

I gulped. I know when I am beaten.

'Not sort of, actually,' I admitted reluctantly.

He sighed. 'Student on a bet, perhaps? Tired of life in the fast lane and looking for a one-way ticket back to the dole queue? Fancy life as a dustman, a postman, or hustling on the streets, maybe?'

'How could you tell?' I asked resignedly.

'Well,' he said, and I swear he wanted to laugh, 'I've been a consultant a long time now, and I've seen nearly everything there is to be seen. And . . . well, they warned me about you in advance. You're Sparrow, aren't you? I've read all your records with some interest.'

I know when I'm beaten. But . . .

I looked at his hand resting quietly on the notes between us in a vague sort of way, barely seeing, scarcely recognizing, and thought to myself, So what's wrong with being a dustman anyway? And couldn't hustling be some sort of fun?

But then my eyes began to focus, and I thought again.

'So what would you do now,' I asked reflectively, 'if you were me, and I you?'

Mr Frankham sat back in his seat, clasped his hands together, and regarded me with some interest.

'Give in gracefully,' he suggested at length. 'Take whatever punishment may be coming your way like a man – it was you leading that riot down the main corridor, wasn't it? – and maybe think about some of those alternative career prospects we discussed earlier.'

But there was a twinkle in his eye that gave me the confidence to push just that little bit further.

'Thank you for your honesty, sir,' I responded. 'But could I trouble you with one last request?'

I almost think he knew what was coming.

'Anything,' he agreed expansively.

'Would you mind holding up your left little finger?' I said quietly.

He did, and I held up mine too. It was hard to be sure which of them was more noticeably bent.

'I have one of those as well,' I continued more equably than I felt, 'although we probably didn't get them in quite the same way. But you tend to notice other people's little anomalies, don't you, sir, when you have something like that yourself? And you see, although you are of course entirely correct in establishing that I'm not strictly speaking an Afro-Caribbean patient with a badly damaged right or left knee, I think I can claim an equal degree of accuracy in stating that I consider it highly unlikely you are really a disgruntled outpatient pretending to start a riot in your own hospital, as such. Are you, sir?'

Mr Frankham sat and regarded me soberly. I stared back, taking in his white coat, his Armani suit and his broken left little finger, and held my breath.

Please God, I prayed silently. Tell me I am right.

And then Mr Frankham, bless him, started laughing, and carried on until the tears began to run down his cheeks. He reached across to the top drawer of his desk and drew out the wig, the glasses, and the tinted contact lenses before laying them out unceremoniously on the desktop blotter between us.

'How much?' he asked solemnly.

'How much what?' I replied, confused.

'How much did they bet you that you could get away with it?'

'Ten pints,' I replied soberly.

'Ten pints,' he sighed, and closed the notes in front of him with a shake of his head. 'Well, one day, Mike – I can call you Mike, can I . . . ?'

'Oh yes, sir,' I reassured him hastily. 'Round about now I think you can call me anything you like.'

' . . . well, one day, Mike, when you get to be as venerably old and excruciatingly bored as I now find myself, you can bet as equally indiscriminately as my esteemed colleagues and myself over events that never fail to be beyond our ultimate control.'

'Could you run to words of two syllables or less?' I begged.

He bit his lip, and leaned forward on the desk. 'I'll make you a deal,' he suggested.

Oh, thank you, God, I thought, saying as nonchalantly as I dared, 'Well, I suppose that depends upon quite what you had in mind.'

'They bet me,' he said slowly, grinning from ear to ear, 'six crates of vintage champagne that I wouldn't get away with it. That is six crates, of our choice of *very* exclusive champagne, may I add.'

'Just the six,' I said faintly.

'Just the six,' he repeated, with a nod of his head. 'And twenty-four bottles to the crate instead of the normal twelve, I suppose I should say. So how would you like to have three of them?'

'And this is very expensive stuff, sir, is it?' I stressed.

'Oh, seriously expensive,' he answered sagely. 'In fact hideously so, if I am to be honest.'

It was probably the single most defining moment of my career.

'I think the one crate, sir, under the circumstances, would be just fine,' I said eventually. 'And then neither of us will feel we have lost out all that much, will we?'

He held out his hand across the desk, and I shook it firmly.

'It's a deal,' he said, grinning expansively, 'as long as you accept two crates and a bottle of my best brandy. And if I may say so, Mike, it has been an unexpected pleasure doing business with you.'

He sat back in his chair and regarded me thoughtfully.

'If you don't mind me saying so,' he said at last, 'I would guess from our most recently shared experiences that there may well be a time or two in your future career as a student when you may be in need of a little helping hand.'

'I think you could be right, sir,' I admitted with a smile.

'My name,' he said, handing me a card, 'out of office hours, is George. I'll be expecting your call . . .'

3

A Spell in Casualty

After finishing my junior house jobs, and before entering the next stage of my career in the RAF, I worked for a spell in the casualty department – a real one, that is, not the unpalatable fictional tripe you generally have served up on television – of a hospital in a large town that had best remain nameless for medico-legal purposes.

One day a thick-set man staggered into the reception area as I happened to be walking past and breathed, 'Diabetic . . . hypo . . . ' before collapsing in a not inconsiderable heap on the floor.

Even I couldn't get this one wrong.

'Diabetes,' I mused reflectively to the nearest available figure in a uniform – until I realized it was a postman who had come in to have a Yorkshire terrier surgically removed from his ankle. 'Come across that one somewhere before, if my memory serves me rightly. But that other word – hypo . . . something? It's a new one on me.'

Casualty nurses are wonderful creatures. Two or three appeared as if by magic, and thirty seconds later one said briskly, 'Blood sugar 2.1,' (very low, 'hypo' actually standing for hypoglycaemia, a potentially dangerous state of low blood sugar most commonly suffered by diabetics on insulin when they have perhaps missed a meal) whilst another slapped a large syringe into my open palm and said, 'Glucose. Patient. Mix together carefully, stand back, and observe.' The third just shook her head in disbelief.

I gave the inert figure on the floor an intravenous injection of that sticky glucose stuff, and stood back, as advised. Low and behold a few short minutes later he recovered, Lazarus-like, metaphorically arising from the dead.

On coming to his senses, however, instead of being overwhelmed with gratitude at our life-saving enterprises, he looked wildly around the department, got to his feet and ran headlong out of the nearest door.

Intrigued by this novel reaction to what I felt was the nearest thing akin to reincarnation, I followed him out into the hospital car park. Patients normally run away before we treat them, if they are going to run away at all, and given some of the long metal implements we wield maliciously in our hands while sidling up to their quaking bodies I, for one, would not generally blame them.

I watched, rooted to the spot in amazement, as he climbed into the cab of one of the largest HGVs I had ever seen and drove off with a screech of brakes. Insulin-dependent diabetics, I should point out, and ruddy great lorries do not usually operate in tandem.

I wandered back thoughtfully into casualty and explained to the waiting staff what had happened.

'What are you going to do?' asked one of the nurses.

'Well,' I replied slowly, 'I took his registration number, and I thought I might give it to you and you might like to ring the police.'

'Me? Why?' she stuttered. 'You can't do that, and nor can I. It's unethical, unprofessional, and against everything we stand for.'

I nodded. 'That may very well be true,' I agreed, 'but I thought you might feel personally involved.'

She regarded me wearily. 'One of your silly games again, Mike?'

'Nope,' I answered sweetly, 'it's just that he happened to crash into the back of your car on the way out.'

Same casualty department, just a couple of days later . . .

I was, for some three years during my time at Lifton, the local police surgeon and was then given pretty clearly defined rules about patient confidentiality. There were strict guidelines about what you could or could not do with information you might obtain during the course of your medical duties, and who you were 'empowered' – I hate that word with a passion exceeding that of my loathing for the Welsh Rugby team – to reveal it to should it be relevant to a particular crime under investigation.

But in the early days of my career it was far from being so succinctly clarified. Like general practice itself things were never clearly delineated as black and white, just an infinite diversity of shades of grey . . .

In the early hours of one Sunday morning I found myself faced with the task of stitching up the wrist and forearm of a wild-eyed young lad who kept looking about him in a distinctly nervous fashion. He had staggered in through the main doors bleeding profusely, clutching a couple of carrier bags in his arms as if his life depended upon them.

You learn, in general, to ask as few questions as possible in casualty, particularly when injuries are involved. It is best just to deal with the medical problem in front of you and let the moral issues involved remain strictly somebody else's domain.

But I was curious, all the same.

'Pop your bags down there,' I suggested. 'They sure as hell won't be going anywhere until you do. Now, come with me and let's have a good look at what you've managed to do to yourself.'

I inspected his wounds under the unforgiving glare of the minor surgery spotlight, whistled softly and surveyed his agitated face.

'I need a few details,' I said quietly. 'Name, address, registered doctor – just for our records,' I reassured him, as he made to get up and go. 'I have to make sure that when I've finished attending to your injuries and sent you ultimately on your way you'll be properly followed up by your own GP.'

He glanced apprehensively again round the department.

'My name's John,' he stuttered hesitantly. 'John – John Smith, that's what it is.'

'Uh huh,' I responded non-committally. 'And I am the proverbial Queen of Sheba . . . No, not really,' I added with a sigh as he looked blankly back at me, 'it's just the sort of mildly amusing but ineffectual witticism we doctors like to make at the expense of the poorly educated lower classes.'

'Like me?' he asked, preening himself in the hermetically sealed HIV resistant casualty mirror as if I had just paid him the ultimate compliment.

'Yes,' I agreed, 'just like you. A prime example of the detritus – sorry, just some archaic medical terminology we generally use for the heavily bleeding patient,' I explained kindly, ' – we so very often encounter here.'

He sat motionless, no doubt awaiting the arrival of an interpreter.

'Well, "John Smith",' I reflected after all due consideration, 'you are currently haemorrhaging profusely all over my casualty floor, and I hate to think of the fuss the cleaners are going to make in the morning. Consider the overtime, and the strain on our dearly beloved NHS that may ultimately ensue. Oh, and don't forget the state of your arm, of course. Shame to be losing it in one so young, after having it live and grow with you so successfully these past seventeen years.'

I peered into his wounds with my best 'Well, it's not my arm so I don't really care too much what happens to it' expression on my face. I was always pretty good at that.

'Oh my,' I continued, after some mock serious deliberation, 'you've gone and done a good one, make no mistake. I could stitch it up for you, I suspect, and make a well above average job of it – had I a mind to. And it's that or amputation, some distance above the elbow . . .' he blanched visibly, much to my satisfaction, ' . . . and I always enjoy the challenge of sawing through bone without the benefit of any local anaesthetic. But I've got a bit of a problem here . . . '

'You have?' squeaked 'John' weakly.

'I have,' I confirmed soberly. 'But by no means as much as yourself. Mine, I feel obligated to relate to you, is referred to in the trade as "short-term memory loss", the same dysfunctional process you appear to have regarding your name. I just cannot at the moment recall how to undertake the restorative surgery you and your arm currently so desperately need.'

'You what?' he asked, appalled

I rested my hand on his shoulder. 'Do you know, John, I am beginning to perceive this horrible feeling that you and your arm might be completely buggered, unless . . . '

It was coffee time, and the doctors' mess was subliminally calling. I came back twenty minutes and a couple of custard creams later as duly refreshed as 'John' was becoming rapidly exsanguinated.

'I have been thinking,' I said slowly, '– a concept you are possibly genetically predetermined to misunderstand – and I reckon I have come across an idea of how to override the little dilemma facing us. I'm beginning to believe that if you were to recall your name, your address, and even the name of your doctor, then I might be able to remember how to stitch up your arm. Of course, if I can't, it will be your arm that will be in need of amputation. I'm sorry,' I admitted, holding my hands out and shrugging, 'but there it is. I just feel honour bound to give you the truth of the situation as I see it – in a genuine, empathic, sharing sort of way, you understand.'

I let it sink in for a moment or two – or at least the shorter words he actually understood – then added carelessly, 'I wonder if you can help me out?'

He nodded, and after a few further minutes of agonizing thought whispered his name.

'Good, Barry,' I enthused. 'I may call you Barry, I hope? Now, if you can remember your address, I might just remember where I left the local anaesthetic. So painful, the sting of the needle on unanaesthetized flesh, and I would feel so unhappy to have to subject you to it. Can you recall your address, Barry? Your real one, that is?'

He nodded again, and recited it slowly for me.

'Good,' I repeated, 'I do believe we're going to get on famously. Now, if you're sitting comfortably – no, don't bleed over that, please, it's one of the nurses and we'll be needing her for other purposes later this evening – then I'll begin.'

I jotted down his details on the casualty card, stuck it in my pocket and then turned my full attention to his injuries. There were some minor scratches around his knuckles, but more importantly two or three quite deep lacerations on his forearm which were bleeding heavily. I whistled softly.

'Nice mess you tried to make of yourself. How did you manage it?'

He looked at me sullenly, and said nothing. Time to take off the velvet gloves.

'Look, young man,' I said harshly, 'I really don't care how you amuse yourself in your spare time – mugging old ladies, watching *Coronation Street* with the sound down or racing stag beetles after hours in the car park of the Dog and Duck – but I need to know how you got these cuts so that I know how to mend them. I need to know if I'm looking for glass in here, or metal, or a complete set of Dobermann's dentures . . . You do understand what I'm saying, don't you?'

He nodded half-heartedly, scarcely trusting himself to speak.

'I'm a doctor,' I continued. 'I'm neither a policeman, a solicitor, nor a woolly-minded liberal social worker who thinks you probably had a hard time in your early life because your father never bonded with you properly and therefore all subsequent behaviour can be excused on a technicality, and I'm sure I like Esther Rantzen even less than you do. I just want to stitch up your wounds to the best of my ability, no matter how undeserving a subject you may be, and make you as healthy in the long run as I am able before the next patient in need of my services comes along to keep me unjustly from my bed and make my already very frayed temper even worse that it currently is. So how did you do this, and bear in mind my patience is very shortly about to run out.'

'Put my arm through a window,' he admitted reluctantly.

'That you had previously neglected to open, I assume. Your own window, or somebody else's – no, on second thoughts, don't bother to answer that. I think I might just possibly be able to tell.'

I carried on stitching in silence for a while, and then, the task completed, stood back to survey my work.

'Nice suturing, Mike,' I congratulated myself, as nobody else seemed about to do it for me. 'A really neat piece of work. Well done.'

My patient looked at me suspiciously. 'Are you for real?' he asked.

'Yup,' I answered. 'As real as those two burly policemen who have just wandered into the casualty department down there, looking for all the world like men with a crime to solve and in search of their suspect.'

'You what?' he burst out, a look of distinct alarm flitting across his weary features, and then coming back and taking up permanent residence. It was soon to be joined by a look of abject panic, the two spending an interesting few moments jostling for prime position.

'I'm just a poor, humble doctor,' I said mildly. 'I do my job, and let everybody else get on with theirs. And the back door is over there,' I pointed obligingly, 'just past the grey-looking chap being sick in the corner.'

He needed no second bidding, and was gone before you could say 'Irish', as in 'Irish stew in the name of the law,' or whatever it is you hear on television, but never in real life.

Of course, the patient had gone, but in his haste he had neglected to realize that behind him was left – amongst other things – his casualty card, still residing in my pocket. I patted it gently, and then slowly followed his line of exit out into the car park, standing there for a few moments whilst I perused the scene thoughtfully. Of 'John Smith' – aka Barry Peter Bonetti – there was no sign.

'Well, Barry, what shall we do about you now?' I murmured to myself, and strolled casually back into the hospital, stopping off at the administration office for a moment.

At that moment, the casualty registrar, Dr Norman, loomed ominously into view. A self-important, busy little man who insisted upon wearing a bow tie on all occasions (practising no doubt for his consultancy, which was irritatingly close to fruition), he had scant time for my less than conventional view of medicine. We were never destined to be the best of friends – I found him to be an obnoxious little git, and he found me mostly in the way.

'Police here, Sparrow,' he said in his clipped fashion. He seemed to abbreviate each word as he addressed his juniors – and lovingly elongated them for his superiors – as if not to waste time or conversation upon us unless absolutely necessary.

'That's nice,' I responded. 'Helmet jammed irretrievably on one of their heads and in need of urgent surgical removal? Manacled themselves together in an idle moment and lost the key? Truncheon . . .'

He glared at me with what I assume he felt was a sufficiently withering manner to deflate a flippant junior, even at 2.30 in the morning.

'They're looking for a couple of kids who have been smashing car windows around here and stealing the radios, and want to know if we can help. Apparently one of them must have cut himself quite badly on a car just outside, and they reckon he must have dashed in here hoping to get himself sorted out before anyone raised the alarm.'

Things were getting interesting. A deliciously taut atmosphere was settling over the department like an early spring mist, although the denouement turned out to be not quite what I was anticipating.

It was not unusual for the police to wander into casualty hoping to fit an injury to a recently perpetrated crime, and we each had our own way of dealing with it. Some merely put up the professional shutters, whereas others all but drove them to the door of the probable suspect and ushered them in.

I was curious to see how Dr Norman would handle the situation, so in the interests of experimentation decided to pass him the buck – lock and stock, if not quite yet smoking barrel.

'Just finished stitching him up, I guess,' I said carelessly. 'Made rather a good job of it too, if I say so myself, twelve stitches at the wrist, twenty-three on the forearm, and a neat little – '

He wasn't too interested in what was neat and little, apparently.

'Casualty card,' he snapped.

'Yes?' I enquired.

'Did you do one, damn it? Or did such a minor detail elude your attention, in your usual haphazard fashion?' He seemed to be getting a touch irritable.

I wrinkled my nose in deep concentration. 'You know, I do believe I did,' I said finally, endeavouring to sound surprised at my unaccustomed efficiency.

'Then give it to me,' he demanded brusquely.

I was beginning to enjoy this. 'Give it to me, *please*,' I corrected, like a primary school teacher admonishing a recalcitrant child.

To his credit, he avoided actually spitting, although I could see the effort involved was exacting a serious toll.

'Give . . . me . . . the casualty card . . . please,' he forced out between clenched teeth, after a few deep breaths and an awful lot of swallowing.

'That's better,' I said approvingly, and passed it across, wondering what plans he might have for it. My curiosity was duly rewarded almost immediately as – not entirely to my surprise – he methodically tore it into the tiniest of little pieces and dropped them with a flourish into the nearest bin. An odious little prig he may have been, but – to give him his credit – he was an ethically odious one. I almost admired him, for a second or two, but caught myself just in time.

'Patient confidentiality is sacrosanct,' he said pompously. 'We cannot be seen to breach the trust they place in us purely because we may privately disapprove of their moral integrity.'

'Humbug,' I muttered under my breath, but he was too busy listening to himself to pay any attention to me.

'You are to say nothing about this matter,' he continued, 'to anyone, under any circumstance, at any time, from this moment onwards. Do you understand?'

'Perfectly,' I replied meekly. 'I will deny any knowledge of this patient and his activities from now on – no matter what the provocation or how just the cause.'

The not-so-subtle hint of sarcasm was entirely lost upon him.

'Good,' he said briskly. 'Good.' And then he regarded me in what I suspect he thought was the manner of a friendly, well-meaning adviser, and laid his hand on my shoulder.

'Well, Sparrow, I think you've learned something here tonight, don't you?'

I think I'm about to, I thought to myself, but merely smiled beatifically and nodded my agreement. 'I do believe I have,' I said seriously, 'and I feel so much the better for it. Now, as it all seems to have quietened down for a while, why don't you take a break and go home? I'll call you if I run into any problems – it will be good for me to take the responsibility for a bit, with the security of knowing you will be there in the background to advise me, should I need it.'

I wondered if I had gone too far, but I needn't have worried. I don't think you could, not with Dr Norman.

'Exactly what I was going to suggest myself,' he said smugly. 'I'll just deal with the police, commiserate and all that and say how sorry we are to be unable to help – not a word, mind . . . '

'Scout's honour,' I agreed solemnly.

' . . . and then I'll be off.'

True to his word, he spoke to the two policemen in his oily 'I'm actually a consultant in all but name and it won't be long before the appointment' manner, collected his coat and walked out into the cold night air.

Thirty seconds, I thought quietly. I'll give him thirty seconds.

Twenty-three seconds later, Dr Norman burst back into the department, wild-eyed and staring.

'Bastard,' he shouted. 'The absolute bloody bastard. It was my bloody car window he cut his bloody arm on and my bloody car radio that's missing.'

A major ethical decision was knocking on my door about now, just begging to be let in.

Dr Norman ran across to where I was sitting and began to search feverishly through the waste paper bin for the scraps of paper he had so diligently torn up, before realizing the ultimate futility of his task.

He glared up at me, red-faced and sweating.

'His name,' he demanded. 'Do you remember his name?'

'I'm not at all sure that I do,' I said nonchalantly. 'There've been so many people through here tonight, and I rarely pay any attention to people's details, to be honest.'

I bit my lip as his face seemed to swell with rage, and turn purple. If only he had been a little nicer to everyone, I might have even felt sorry for him, which was a shame, really, because . . . well, because underneath the desk in front of me my foot was resting on a certain pair of carrier bags Barry had left behind in his haste. And in my other pocket was the photocopy of the casualty card I had taken on my brief stop in the admin office.

'I think,' I said finally, entirely without inflection, watching with some interest as his breathing become ever more laboured by the second, 'I think that we have both learned something here tonight. Haven't we?'

Of course, telling the undiluted truth may have a gloriously moralistic cleansing effect, but sometimes there are unforeseen – and occasionally regrettable – consequences.

I was sitting in the office one day when one of the nurses entered the department and called across to me.

'Hey, Mike, what happened to Mr Kelsey?'

I thought carefully. 'Was that the chap in cubicle three with a cricket ball in a place you wouldn't normally encounter one?'

'No, not him,' she replied with a grin spreading across her mischievously dimpled face, 'we all know what happened to *him*. No, the man in cubicle six with the arthritic knee?'

'Ah, him,' I answered, wincing. 'Well, unfortunately for all concerned Dr Atherton mistook him for Mr McMichaels – you know, the bloke in cubicle five who had just had a cardiac arrest – and rushed in and shoved the defibrillator on his chest whilst he was having a quiet doze waiting to go down to X-ray. Mr McMichaels failed to have his heart restarted, but we consoled ourselves with the fact that he was eighty-six and had little chance of survival in any case, and he's now dead.'

'Oh my God,' she breathed.

'It gets worse,' I warned. 'More unfortunately than that, Mr Kelsey – whose heart was probably good for another ten to fifteen years under normal circumstances – failed to successfully nego-tiate a 400 joule shock from a defibrillator he didn't explicitly need, and now he's dead too. The undertaker's been informed, of course – we didn't want to bother the coroner, poor chap has so much work on his plate as it is – and said that was quite OK because he could pick up two for the price of one and he'll be along within the hour.'

Every word of which was sadly true. I wonder, looking back, what we might have done had events not forced our hand. Quietly pretend nothing had happened? Well, yes, quite possibly, as mainly – true to the normal traditions of medicine – there but for the grace of God went all the rest of us. Catastrophic mistakes are so easy to make when you are tired, emotionally strung out, and lacking in the necessary professional capabilities.

But all was very far from equal. Mr Kelsey's wife and daughter were understandably curious to discover what had happened to their respective husband and father. He had after all only ventured into casualty with a bad knee, and left with pretty much a bad everything. Unbeknownst to myself they had burst into the department on a voyage of discovery just as I started talking, and were standing right behind my left shoulder.

You would not have thought the situation could get any worse, could you? But it did . . . as what ultimately ended Dr Atherton's career and the lives of Mr Kelsey and Mr McMichaels tragically accounted for Mrs Kelsey, as well. On becoming inadvertently acquainted with the awful news she collapsed on the spot from a fatal heart attack, all our best endeavours failing to revive her.

If you should think, upon reading this now some twenty years after the above events, that my attitude exhibited a degree of callousness far beyond that which is in any way forgivable, then in many respects I would have to agree with you.

But what you must understand is that in a young doctor's career life and death come and go as indiscriminately as children in a sweet shop. We have to learn to adjust to the inevitability of undeserved departure from this mortal coil of ours, and find a way to be unmoved by it in order to survive. One of the first lessons to comprehend is that no matter how hard we may try patients will always die for no better reason than because sometimes they do, and they will, and on occasion may even want to.

Life, dare I say it, is unaccountably like that. As soon as one person has died and is beyond our help there is always someone else who comes along in desperate need of our assistance. We have to learn to control our emotions for the sake of the next patient, and the one after that.

Without wishing in any way to offend anyone who has taken an overdose when in the depths of genuine despair, I have to say that the almost universal response of any junior physician or casualty officer I have ever met on learning there is an overdose heading their way is 'Oh God, not another one.'

This is not primarily because we are hard-bitten, cynically uncaring cybernauts (they all go into hospital administration) but because 'We Know What That Means.'

It means a stomach washout.

Now, I have absolutely no idea what it does to the patient, and quite frequently I could not care less, but I do know what it does to the doctor as you pour pint after pint of lukewarm water into their stomachs and then watch pint after pint flow back in front of you – into a bowl, if you are lucky – together with most of the contents of their last meal. And Billy Connolly is right – it always, but always, contains diced carrots, even when they haven't eaten any for weeks.

'Will I die, doctor?' they tend to gasp between retches.

'Hopefully,' I would mutter viciously, wondering whether the casualty sister or myself would be the first to start vomiting in sympathy.

Amazingly, some patients seemed to be addicted to stomach washouts. Honestly. I can understand most addictions, particularly the nicotine / caffeine / alcohol combination, and I have always been particularly drawn to pork pies and Smarties. I can even understand the attraction for some of colonic lavage, about which I could, but won't, append a very rude joke (it being impossible to append a clean one), but stomach washouts? Some things defy the imagination.

Week after week they would come back, an evil glint in their eye.

'It's paracetamol, this time, doctor, thirty-nine and a half – should have been forty but the last one was all crumbly and I dropped some of the bits on the floor. I suppose this means a washout, doctor?' they would add excitedly.

I'm sure some of them must have been health service employees in the Professional Torturers department, a clandestine segment of that inaugust body designed purely to inflict the maximum discomfiture on as many junior staff as they are able in as limited a timespan as is humanly possible. They were probably on at least double our hourly rate, and given our respective duties no doubt good value for it, too. After each session I expect they would retire to a secret destination and evaluate our performance, giving marks out of ten for ashenness of colour, amount splashed on the floor, number of times fainted . . .

Inevitably, one day, I just cracked.

In response to the ubiquitous 'I suppose this means a stomach washout, doctor?' from one of our regulars, I responded bluntly, 'No, it bloody well doesn't,' and turned to move on to the next patient.

A look of genuine alarm began to spread across his face.

'But that means . . . if you don't do it . . . I could . . . I might *die*,' he said, aghast.

'Isn't that the general idea,' I asked mildly, 'of taking an overdose? You obviously want to kill yourself, having tried so often yet so sadly unsuccessfully, so I thought this time I would accede to your wishes. Instead of consistently denying you the chance to carry out your avowed intent, I'm going to let you get on with it. A doctor's duty is to help their patient live the life they choose – in your case currently a pretty short one – and I'm sorry I've failed to give you the chance to end it before. I have been remiss in my duty, and have resolved not be so remiss any more.'

And I walked away, leaving him there, panicking.

'By the way,' I added as an afterthought, 'try not to worry. If it doesn't work this time, I'm willing to give you another chance.'

In case you are wondering, no, he didn't die on this occasion, having probably taken only the nine and a half paracetamol, and neglected to shovel down the remaining thirty.

But he never came back, either . . .

However, even my world-weary, hard-bitten cynicism – sorry, cool professional detachment – could be melted on occasion.

I was working away as diligently as ever – testing the blood pressure monitors to see just how far you could blow them up before they exploded, and whether you could speed up the process by jumping on them whilst they were three-quarters inflated – when the casualty sister called across to me.

'Mike – sorry to interrupt your highly technical research . . . overdose, cubicle two. And go easy on her,' she pleaded, 'please. None of your "Well, if you really want to do it properly" routines. She's just a kid, and she's so frightened. OK?'

'OK,' I agreed absently, with absolutely no intention of doing anything of the sort.

The casualty sister knew me well. 'You've no intention of doing anything of the sort,' she said sternly. 'Have you?'

I shook my head. 'None,' I agreed. 'None whatsoever. Being nice to the emotionally inadequate is not in my contract.'

'Nor is wheeling the intensive care patients out on to the balcony for a cigarette,' she reminded me. 'But that's never stopped you, has it?'

I admit to cowardice in the face of a strong woman, especially when the strong woman in question held the key to the only broom cupboard large enough to fit two people with the door closed at one and the same time.

'She's sweet,' she continued. 'You'll like her.' And as I turned away I swear she murmured to the blood-soaked dressing she was in the process of changing, 'Mmmm, nice congealed jelly bits on the outside, Mrs Pilkington,' as if she was judging the best fairy cake at the village fete, before calling back to me, 'Though whether she'll like you, of course, is a different matter . . .'

And she *was* sweet. I *did* like her. Just sixteen, doe eyes brimming with tears staring up at me, bottom lip quivering as if it would never stop – had she been my daughter I would have locked her in the basement for a good ten years, and then probably another ten after that.

'I had a row with my mum,' she sobbed, 'and . . . and I've taken too many of these. I didn't mean to, I really didn't, and I'm so sorry for any trouble I've caused. Am I going to die?'

I looked at the bottle she held out to me, and bit my lower lip. 'How many of these have you taken, Anna?' I asked gently.

'Three,' she burst out, her voice beginning to break, 'and all together, too. Oh, I didn't mean to, I wish my mum was here. What's going to happen to me?'

She was so convinced she was going to die, my heart went out to her. Luckily, however, despite my years of stultifying inactivity at medical school, together with the woeful lack of information it had imparted in my general direction, I had the sneaking suspicion that she might actually live. Three tablets of penicillin are most unlikely to kill an otherwise healthy sixteen-year-old girl, unless she were to trip over them at the top of a very tall flight of concrete steps.

'Well, Anna,' I began, 'what's going to happen now is . . .'

And then something unaccountable took place, something I can still not explain after all these years.

What I thought I was going to say was, 'Well, what's going

to happen now is that I shall get a very large and unsympathetic casualty sister to wash your stomach out, a process only marginally more enjoyable than being disembowelled with a very blunt instrument. After that, we will admit you to the psychiatric ward with all the real nutters as a potential suicide risk and leave you in complete darkness while they howl and slobber somewhere near the end of your bed. Then all sorts of really unpleasant people will come and question you about your childhood and whether anyone has ever really loved you at any stage of your life, and finally tomorrow we shall publish your name, address and photograph in all the local papers with the heading "Anyone know this underachieving fruitcake? Please come and get her from the funny farm — protective clothing advised." And if that doesn't stop you wasting my precious time in the future, and denying my services to patients who are really ill and not just pathetically attention-seeking, then what I'll be doing next is . . . '

It usually works pretty well by this point, the younger ones lying there gibbering until I unroll the straitjacket, but on this occasion it just wouldn't come out. I tried, and I tried again, but it was no good.

'Well, Anna,' I said in a voice I could not entirely recognize as my own — it having compassion in it, 'what's going to happen now is that you and I are going to go and ring your mum, and tell her you are fine and you just want to go home, and could she possibly come and get you. Is that all right with you?'

'Yes,' she snivelled endearingly, 'oh yes, please. But am I going to die after that?'

'Eventually,' I smiled, 'because we all will, one day, but not because of this.' I pursed my lips, considering. 'I should think that you're good for another sixty years or so, judging it on the conservative side.'

She looked at me then as if I was the most wonderful man in the world, and probably even the universe, and for one small moment I began to understand what the word 'vocation' really meant.

'I don't have any money for the phone,' she said in a small voice.

'But luckily I do,' I replied. 'Come on, Anna, off we go. Your mum will be getting worried. But don't tell any of the nurses I was nice to you, will you? I could never look them in the face again if they began to suspect that beneath this badly fitting white coat there is a heart beating, somewhere.'

So Anna, wherever you now are, I hope life has treated you kindly, and that you have never been as unhappy again as on the one day we met all those years ago. I would also just like to point out that you managed to ruin my hard-earned reputation for callousness beyond the call of duty, for ever – in that hospital, at least.

After she had left, with her mother's arms wrapped protectively around her, I wandered back to casualty, feeling unaccustomedly happy. The casualty sister walked over to where I sat smoking a reflective cigarette, and considered me carefully.

'Goodness,' she said at last. 'I do believe it has a heart. Always thought it must have, somewhere or other, but never thought we ever would see it, and so clearly, too.'

And to my great surprise she bent over and kissed me on the cheek before wandering off down the corridor carrying something unmentionable over her shoulder, saying, 'Just wait till I tell the others. They'll never believe a word of it.'

For all the above incidents, casualty could sometimes be a quiet, humdrum, unexciting place. On these occasions my day could often be enlivened by the odd trip to the wards.

'Mike,' phoned Mark, one of the junior housemen, urgently. 'Help! It's Mr Hutchinson.'

'Which Mr Hutchinson?' I asked, as if the entire hospital was crammed full of Hutchinsons, spilling out into the corridors and overflowing through the front entrance into the hospital car parks.

'Ward 14, grey hair, came in through casualty today for investigation of abdominal pain . . . you saw him . . . '

'Rings no bells,' I admitted doubtfully.

' . . . shoved his hand up Matron's skirt and claimed it was an involuntary muscular spasm?'

'Ah, *that* Mr Hutchinson,' I acknowledged. 'He with the less than discriminatory taste and bilateral cataracts. Even the chap in the next bed, you know, Mr Philips with the total body failure, said the only thing that should be in Matron's skirt was Matron's legs, and given the choice even they would probably rather be somewhere else. By the way, have you heard —'

'Mike, for goodness sake, I'm desperate . . . '

'You must be if you're ringing me,' I agreed.

' . . . and it's your help I was wanting, not the latest bit of hospital gossip, so please get your backside over here as fast as you can — he's having some odd sort of fit, Ali' (as everyone called his registrar, whose name was unpronounceably longer) 'is stuck in a meeting somewhere and I don't have the first clue what to do with him.'

A few minutes later I too stood at the end of Mr Hutchinson's bed . . .

'Ooh, look, he's having some kind of fit,' I observed brightly.

. . . and I too did not know what to do with him.

'Any ideas?' asked Mark desperately.

'Well,' I opined seriously, 'strikes me we have just two choices here.'

'As many as two?' he replied, raising his eyebrows in mock surprise.

'Yup, that many. Number one — run away quickly and try to pretend we haven't noticed anything amiss. Number two — panic a bit, ask for lots of expensive machinery and investigations, and start sticking needles in him like crazy, with drugs and things, like real doctors do.'

He pursed his lips thoughtfully. 'Good appraisal, Mike. I rather like the running away option, myself, but do you think any of these good nurses here, or the other twenty-six patients on the ward, might notice if we did?'

'Only if he needed witnesses,' I replied firmly, 'and there was money involved.'

'"Junior doctors run away from patient having a fit", you mean,' said Mark, anticipating the headlines. '"Student nurse says "I knew he was really ill but they just wouldn't listen to me." And how about "Long-lost mother grieves for son she never knew.""'

'You should have had a job with the tabloids,' I said admiringly.

The nurse to my right coughed pointedly. 'I do so hate to interrupt your private conversation,' she said, 'but don't you think you had better do something about Mr Hutchinson instead of merely working on your comedy routine? He's not looking all that well.'

We looked at Mr Hutchinson, and considered. She was right – he wasn't looking at all well, and was getting progressively worse by the second.

'Right,' said Mark decisively, 'I think I've got it sorted. You run around and panic for a bit, I'll call for the expensive machinery, and then we'll do what proper doctors do on the telly, and we don't.'

'And what's that?' I demanded.

'Oh, discuss interesting cases, drive expensive cars, dress for ward rounds like you're going out for dinner and employ Hungarian nannies to look after the golden retriever and those still quiet hours of the morning when the wife is away doing good works. And there's something else . . . what is it now? No, don't tell me, it'll come to me in a moment . . .'

'Have affairs with the nurses?'

'Don't be silly — we can do that as well,' he added scornfully. 'No, hang on ... it's coming ... I've got it! Treat people appropriately to their needs.'

'Gosh,' I said, 'you've done this before, haven't you?'

'Many times,' he agreed, a little pompously, before adding with complete honesty, 'but never successfully.'

The nurse, our collective conscience, coughed even more pointedly than before.

'What is it with you two?' she asked. 'Are you in training for the Christmas panto, or something? Do something verging on the therapeutic, for goodness sake. Something soon.'

Of course, you are thinking to yourselves, doctors don't really talk like this at the end of a patient's bed during a time of deepening medical crisis. Do they?

I'm afraid that they do.

It's our defence mechanisms at work. It is how we get through those desperate, uncertain moments when we feel apprehensive and alone, unequal to the task facing us and uncertain how to proceed. It's how we cope with the inevitable loss of life, the shuddering jolt of a catastrophic mistake, the automatic all-night chocolate machine running out of change ...

Mr Hutchinson was now turning worryingly grey.

His hands were locked in tetanic spasm, his breathing was shallow and laboured and his hold on life precipitously tenuous. Suddenly our light-hearted flippancy seemed very much out of place. Our patient looked as if he was about to die, and to be honest we were totally unsure how we were going to deal with it.

We frantically did all the doctoring bits we could think of, gave him most of the available drugs at our disposal ... and nothing happened. A sense of impending doom was spreading around us, and even the patients in the nearby beds were beginning to sense our rapidly developing impotence as we stood there, hearts in our mouths, waiting for something cataclysmic to happen and yet hoping so fervently it would not.

Suddenly a voice spoke behind us.

'OK, Mr Hutchinson, you can stop all this now.'

We turned abruptly to see the gently smiling face of Ali behind us.

'You can stop it now, Mr Hutchinson,' he repeated lightly in his sing-song voice. 'You've been grumbled.'

'I think you mean rumbled,' I whispered.

'You might mean rumbled, but I'm sticking with grumbled,' said Ali, beaming now from ear to ear. 'I'm Indian, so I can humorously mispronounce your language as much as I like, and we can all laugh about it later. So stop pretending to have a fit, Mr Hutchinson,' he continued, an ominous undercurrent in his voice, 'stop taking up a hospital bed that someone who is seriously ill could use so much more efficiently than you, and start getting ready to make your way home before I call for the soap and water enemas.'

We turned back to Mr Hutchinson, transfixed. Miraculously, before our very eyes, he stopped fitting instantaneously, returned to his normal colour – still not a particularly pretty one, but a distinct improvement on the one he'd been giving us for the past twenty minutes – sat up, and started breathing normally.

'Now then, Mr Hutchinson,' admonished Mark, wagging his finger so ferociously in his direction that even I was impressed, 'don't you be doing that again or you'll have me to answer to,' and we trailed off meekly in Ali's wake.

'Don't be doing what?' I asked, half-way down the corridor.

'Haven't the faintest idea,' he admitted, 'I just wanted to look like I knew what I was doing, for a moment.'

It was that supreme sense of control, in a time of apparent crisis, that made such an impression. Some day, I thought forlornly, I would actually understand a bit of medicine, too.

We sat in the nurses' office, Ali still smiling serenely away at some huge joke only he seemed to understand. We just had to ask.

'How did you do that?' Mark and I chorused together.

Ali opened his mouth, still grinning broadly, and uttered but one word.

There is a disease now far more widely known amongst both the general public and practitioners due to several high profile cases of recent times, but of which nearly twenty years ago I was scarcely aware — save for a few inconsequential lines in the most voluminous of medical textbooks. It is a disease where patients pretend to be seriously ill for their own ends, frequently resulting in major treatments or operations for conditions that do not exist. If you have never seen it, and sometimes even if you have, it can be almost unrecognizable, and far better doctors than Mark and myself have been fooled by the more proficient protagonists.

But once seen in this form, it is never forgotten.

'Munchausen's,' said Ali, shrugging nonchalantly.

The doctor's white coat has a great deal to answer for — sometimes rather more than you might think.

It has, for a start, a significant effect both on those within it, and on those without. There is, for example, a benign medical condition known as 'White Coat Hypertension'. This now well-recognized phenomenon causes the patient's blood pressure to rise alarmingly the minute they walk into a doctor's surgery, or a hospital, only to revert to normal the moment they manage to get themselves out again, fleeing as far away as possible in the opposite direction.

We so often treat these patients inappropriately aggressively, bound by the demands of our autocratically dictated governmental protocols rather than the intrinsic needs of our patient. Because that, as we are so constantly reminded, is the way our duty is deemed to lie.

More sinister by far, however, is the 'White Coat Syndrome', a nasty, pernicious disease that affects a particularly unpleasant sub-species of society – generally the person inside it. Even the humblest, most God-fearing of medical students may disturbingly transform into a dictator amongst men when donning for the first time the long white coat . . . all the better for striding down the corridors in.

You can easily assess the knowledge, professionalism and all-round general medical ability of any doctor from the white coat they wear, or more accurately the amount of paraphernalia they have crammed into their various pockets. There is an inverse law of proportions at work here – the more books, stethoscopes, auroscopes, patella hammers and tuning forks you carry around with you, the less you actually know.

Me? I used to put all the equipment I needed in a supermarket trolley and push it around the wards in front of me. When the wheels finally buckled and gave way I realized it was time to give up the unequal struggle and take the only possible way out.

I became a GP, moved out to the countryside and bought a Volvo. You can get an awful lot of paraphernalia in a Volvo.

Casualty departments are full of white coats. Long ones, short ones, clean and grubby ones . . . white coats that belong there and white coats that do not, but are just passing through.

My colleagues and I had an ingeniously simple protocol for survival. Fill the casualty department with as many white coats as you could find – preferably some of them with doctors in – and consequently make it as difficult as possible for anyone to know whom to blame when it all went completely 'Pete Tong'.

I think we may have taken things too far when, one quiet evening with no accumulated group of patients to maltreat for a couple of hours, we emblazoned on the wall of the casualty department in six foot high letters: 'It's not our fault. You could have gone somewhere else.'

But it seemed like an awfully good idea at the time.

The six casualty officers in the department worked 'round the clock' shifts – twenty-four hours on, twenty-four hours off and twenty-four hours trying to remember where your family lived, and what their names were – under the benign tutelage of two registrars with genetically inherited Attention Deficit Disorders, a prerequisite for the post. Above them was the intellectually challenged 'Overlord' masquerading as the consultant in charge, despite being blessed with all the innate charm of Vlad the Impaler, though without any of his redeeming features.

At the start of work each day we would drag ourselves to his office for what we called 'the mourning round', whereupon he would nobly and self-sacrificingly run through a list of our failings, collective or otherwise, from the previous day, and then run through them again. Should time allow (and strangely, it never once seemed to) he would then praise us warmly for our successes, and speak glowingly of us to his friends, neighbours and casual acquaintances.

'Didn't drain that tension pneumothorax' (collapsed lung) 'before they got it out of the ambulance, then, Sparrow? Patient could have died, man, and then what would you have done?'

I never did learn. 'Well, nothing, sir, if he was dead. Wouldn't have been much point then, would there?'

Or 'Davies – how many times have I told you never, never, *never* to undertake a rectal examination on a suspected ectopic pregnancy beyond the confines of the operating theatre and without the presence of a gynaecological team all gowned up, and ready to go?'

'Um, never, sir,' said Davies with a thoughtful look on his face. 'Until now, that is.'

Attila, as we endearingly called him, was always meticulously dressed, being invariably attired in a white coat that seemed never to have encountered a single bodily exudate.

You might occasionally catch him working, however, incising

abcesses without the benefit of an anaesthetic or removing an ingrowing toenail with a maniacal look in his eye.

The casualty department had four rows of cubicles, five in each row. On their arrival, patients – were they both literate and conscious, not all that common a combination in that part of the world – would be given a card to fill out, and each of these was placed in chronological order to be picked up by the next available casualty officer. Emergencies were dealt with as and when they arose.

As doctors we often carried several cards around with us at any one time, juggling the patients and cubicle-hopping according to need. This would depend to some extent on the degree of medical urgency, but more importantly on how pretty the nurse with the patient was.

You could hear the constant cries of 'Fractured pelvis in cubicle four – I need an orthopod, please,' above the general uproar, or 'Enema cubicle seven, please, and naso-gastric tube cubicle twelve – and don't get them mixed up!'

I even once heard the aforementioned Davies call to the casualty sister at the desk, 'I've got a syringe full of narcan here,' (the antidote to an overdose of morphine) 'and I'm looking for a patient to give it to.'

'Try cubicle three,' she yelled back, 'or failing that, four, six or nine in that order. If they're all empty, just shove it into anyone you come across who's asleep in the department. Apart from Attila, that is, who seems to have just nodded off in his office. Poor man – seen four whole patients in the same afternoon and hasn't managed to inflict any unnecessary suffering on a single one of them. Plum tuckered out, he is, from all that lack of torturing. He'll be suffering an acute case of withdrawal tomorrow – better watch out for the "mourning" round.'

It was a dreadful afternoon and evening, one of the worst I can recall, with a succession of major problems interspersed with the usual interminable minor ones, not to mention the even more interminable variety of 'shouldn't have been there in the first place'. Sorting the seriously ill from the seriously time-wasting can be an impossible task, and mistakes will inevitably happen.

Earaches may be seen before heart attacks, minor lacerations before serious head injuries, head colds before overdoses. It is neither easily defensible nor anyone's prime responsibility, which sadly does not mean that when something goes horribly wrong everyone is not looking for somebody else to blame.

'It wasn't my fault,' you could hear people muttering in their quiet moments, practising for the day it would be needed, 'I'd only just come on duty,' or 'I was having a cup of tea at the time.'

I was due off shift at midnight, but it was not until 2.30 in the morning that I eventually crawled into my bed and slept fully clothed, too exhausted to undress. Even Attila had been working away until midnight, a hitherto unheard-of occurrence.

The telephone rang, and rang and rang until I answered it.

'Mike . . . Mike!' said a voice urgently. 'It's Carol, from casualty. Major crisis – just get here quick, will you,' and the line went dead.

I did not need to dress, due to the combination of fatigue and my phenomenal evening's work rate the night before. It had, of course, nothing at all to do with the four double gins I had demolished as quickly as I could pour them on returning to my room, being in need of a little relaxation after a long and difficult day. I rushed immediately down to the casualty department with that sinking feeling we all knew so well, to find Attila, impeccably besuited as usual but for once without his white coat, prowling the corridor outside his office with death in his eyes.

'You're the last,' he hissed. 'My office. Now.'

Unusually I had no sardonic response to hand, but quietly did as I was bidden. I entered his office where all the available casualty staff were already assembled, shifting uneasily from foot to foot.

'What gives?' I murmured to Davies.

'Heard of the warpath?' he whispered back. 'He's just reinvented it.'

The office fell suddenly quiet as Attila entered, looking more ominously menacing than usual, were that possible. We all waited, and the tension grew steadily until at last he spoke.

'Cubicle twenty,' he began. 'Can anybody tell me about cubicle twenty?'

It must have been the tension that brought it out of me.

'Magnolia walls, partly torn curtain, down at the end on the right,' I offered genially. 'Would you like me to show you?'

He looked at me as if I had just crawled out of a gutter, and for a second I rather wished I had.

'Cubicle twenty,' he spat out again. 'At 3.15 yesterday afternoon Mr James Aldridge, an eighty-five-year-old man with a minor stomach ailment, entered the department. We know that because he is logged into the casualty book, but there is no card for him, and nobody appears to remember seeing him – until 7.25 this morning, that is, when one of the cleaners found him dead in the cubicle.'

The room remained completely quiet, even Davies looking pale and somewhat interesting.

'They tell me,' continued Attila, 'that he had been dead for at least twelve hours, possibly more. So what I want to know . . . ' he paused, obviously choosing his words carefully, 'what I want to know is, which of your careers is about to come to an abrupt and unpleasantly painful end?'

We all looked around, searching for guilty faces in the hope that it might be somebody else and then feeling awful for the thought. I sank my hands in the strangely empty pockets of my white coat, and the room began to swim and hum before my eyes as one of them alighted on a piece of card. Slowly, my heart pounding, I drew out the casualty record card of the dead man in cubicle twenty and held it out wonderingly for all to see.

There was a collective intake of breath as we all looked at it, unable to remove our eyes from the terrible truth resting so neatly in my trembling hand. I looked up slowly and met the heavy-lidded gaze of Attila. I would swear that he was smiling, smiling through the sheer awfulness of it all.

'And how, Dr Sparrow,' he said harshly, 'do you think you would like to explain this to the rest of us?'

The rest of them waited, and I thought, and then waited some more. My career, yet again, was beginning to drop down the yawning chasm rapidly opening in front of me. And then:

'Cubicle twelve,' whispered Davies urgently in my ear, 'the man in cubicle twelve,' and the chasm began to close almost as quickly as it had opened.

'Davies, I love you,' I murmured back as Attila said evilly, 'We are waiting, Dr Sparrow. Talk to us while you still have a qualification to your name.'

'Well, it was the chap in cubicle twelve, sir,' I said slowly, feeling my way carefully through the minefield, 'with the bleeding varicose veins at about one o'clock this morning. Bled everywhere, he did, over the sheets, the walls, the floor, Sister Dimonica and . . . and over my white coat, sir. Covered in it, I was, and I know, sir, how you like us to look smart in the department so I took it off, put it out for the laundry and picked up the nearest one to hand . . . Nice suit you have on, sir. Never seen you in the department without your white coat on before . . . '

And we all looked on as Attila sagged down in his chair, suddenly grey, and sank his head into his hands.

4

Doctors, Dentists and Bob

'So what made you join the RAF?' my friends used to ask. 'You don't exactly appear to have been ideally suited.'

'How observant,' I would mutter sardonically beneath my breath. 'And how sadly lacking in originality . . .'

'And what,' generally followed shortly afterwards, 'was it that made you leave?'

It's been a not very closely guarded secret until now, but for those of you unacquainted with the facts, here goes . . .

Having survived the rigorous, in-depth interview (see *Country Doctor: Tales of a rural GP*) during which my need to sign on the dotted line was vastly outweighed by their need to get anyone, anyone at all, to expand the diminishing ranks of junior RAF doctors, I was offered the prize I most wanted.

'Well, Dr Sparrow, I have to tell you that you have been accepted,' smiled the Group Captain grimly, through gritted teeth. 'You can pick up your celebratory bag of dolly mixtures on the way out.'

'Yippee,' I crowed triumphantly.

'But there is one more thing,' continued the Group Captain. 'It is all subject to the medical, of course. You will be sent an appointment for a twenty-four-hour stay at Biggin Hill within a month or two.'

'Is that fairly stringent, sir?' I asked, slightly concerned, aware that a long-standing back injury might cloud my future prospects.

'Just turn up sober,' he sighed, with an imperceptible shake of his head. 'On the right day, at the right time, and with no incumbent parasitic infections. The Air Force needs you, Dr Sparrow.'

'Even if nobody else does,' added his colleague, rather unkindly.

It was an odd experience, arriving at Biggin Hill. Like the interview, nothing I encountered seemed to be quite real. It was as if the whole thing was drafted along the lines of one of those endless television reconstructions we are so often subjected to these days. Everything is more or less as it should be until you remember that all the participants are bit-part actors playing a role, and the minute the camera stops filming they all revert to normality.

Perhaps it was just having spent a year in the smouldering cauldron of the outside world, suddenly to return to what felt like an overgrown kindergarten. For everyone there seemed to be a childlike entity encapsulated in a Disney-like bubble world, where everything is nice, and clean, and well-mannered, and Bambi's mother is doomed forever to die off screen, without any visible bloodshed.

To my surprise I was the only doctor present amongst a small number of potential administration, engineering and air traffic control officers, but we were vastly outnumbered by the staggering array of prospective pilots. I knew full well that I would pass the medical – they needed me, for goodness sake – and anyway, if a doctor couldn't pull the wool over their eyes with respect to a potentially dodgy back, then who on earth could?

I duly sailed, as anticipated, through the various examinations without incident, blithely unpressurized and at first wondering what all the fuss was about. But then, as my passage into the next stage of my career became routinely assured, I began to sit back and take stock of my surroundings and my fellow compatriots.

Amazingly, there was not a single woman to be seen. All around me, instead, were young men barely old enough to shave who were so desperate to be accepted into the RAF that it made me almost (but not quite!) ashamed to be so cavalier about it.

I was by this time, I should point out, a battle-hardened veteran of twenty-five. Having – like all those I sweated blood with throughout the marathon years of medical school – been forged in the iron furnace of academic endeavour, I had then been battered beyond the point of exhaustion by the indisputably inhuman existence that junior hospital doctors had then to endure. Goodness, now I come to describe it I realize that I had quite forgotten what a miserable experience we had been subjected to. Perhaps I can still sue.

But on further reflection there was little of life I hadn't seen – on the wards, during the overnight shift of a weekend duty in casualty or more disturbingly round the back of the nurses' quarters in the early hours of a Sunday morning.

I had to constantly remind myself that these keenly enthusiastic applicants surrounding me were in fact just boys – seventeen- and eighteen-year-olds whose whole life at the time seemed to them to be hanging in the balance of a hearing test, a potential heart murmur, a past history of asthma. As each hour passed another would fall by the wayside, and I began to feel guilty. Why was it that I – who basically cared not a jot what might next happen – should sail through everything unscathed, secure in the knowledge that my immediate future was assured, whilst they, on the other hand, who cared so passionately about their ultimate survival, were subject to what in many ways seemed to me to be the whim of ageing and irrelevant RAF doctors who knew as much about medicine as I did about the correct protocol for attendance at Buckingham Palace garden parties?

I kept to myself, for the most part, feeling uncomfortably like an outsider until the station bar on the second night of my stay was poised to close at the unrealistic hour of ten o'clock. The door swung open.

'Off to bed with you now,' announced the smug, self-satisfied junior officer who had just entered, a man with apparently as much life experience as a battery hen but without the accompanying street credibility.

The room rapidly cleared, leaving only myself and John, a young lad of barely eighteen, sharing a pint together in the now all but deserted bar.

'Shall we move on?' I suggested. 'As a matter of necessity . . . '

'Move on?' he said, startled. 'But he just told us . . . move on where?' he added, narrowing his eyes as the prospect suddenly began to appeal.

'To anywhere that might be open,' I expounded, 'out there in the real world. Like a pub, for example, a lap dancing club, or maybe a late night gambling emporium?'

But this was Biggin Hill. The pub it was.

Unlike so many of the others I had briefly met, John, my new-found companion, had a sense of ironic humour lurking behind his juvenile enthusiasm. He had breezed through the first day of medicals and apparently excelled at the hand-eye co-ordination techniques so vital for prospective pilots.

'It's what I've dreamt about for years,' he explained simply. 'It's what my whole world has revolved around for as long as I can remember. But you, Mike – and I know I don't know you properly, or anything, and I don't mean to be disrespectful, but I get the feeling that if you didn't get through all this you would just shrug your shoulders and say, "Oh well, on to the next thing." I don't think it would matter to you in the same way it would to me.'

'You're right,' I agreed, motioning to the barman for another drink. 'Of course you're right, because we come from different worlds, different perspectives. But John . . . look, I have to say this, because medicine is what I do for a living, have you considered that it might not work out the way you originally planned it?'

'No,' he said determinedly, 'not at all. It's what I want, it's what I've always wanted. And I know, if not before now then just from today, that I have the aptitude, the concentration, I've passed all the co-ordination tests with flying colours . . . I can do this, I know I can. I know I can . . . '

'But John,' I said, not knowing quite how to proceed, 'you do realize that – ?'

'Where's that drink you were talking about then?' he asked, changing the subject. 'Or is that a silly question?'

The survivors from the first day had but a couple of further investigations to undergo. For me, and my recall is not what it was, I think it was a hearing test, a chest X-ray and maybe a final urine sample, but we all had our different rotas.

'Yes, you've passed,' said a world-weary sergeant half-way through the morning. 'But then you would do, sir, wouldn't you, even if you weren't as fit as the proverbial fiddle?'

I went up to my room, packed my bags and made my way back down to reception to sign out, glad to be leaving. After all the uncertainties of the past year this was at last one day when I knew where I was heading. Half-way across the compound to the car park I spotted John sitting forlornly on a bench beneath a huge yew tree on the edge of the drive.

'They turned me down,' he said, tears welling in his eyes as I walked across to him. 'And on the very last test, too. I just can't believe they could do that to me.'

'Neither can I,' I sympathized, scarcely knowing what to say. 'Oh, John, I tried to warn you, last night, but . . . '

'But I didn't want to listen, did I?' He turned away, looking back over the valley, his shoulders sagging with despair. 'How could I have been so stupid, Mike? How could I have failed to see what was staring me so obviously in the face?'

'Oh, John,' I said, struggling to find the right words. 'It wasn't you, not you at all. It's them — how could they have been so lacking in thought and foresight, so unfair . . ?'

He had done everything — IQ testing, co-ordination techniques, heart-lung-stamina procedures, pogo-sticking . . . everything that could ever have been required of him. Until the final test — which could, which should in his case have been the very first, and maybe the only one.

'I failed on my eyesight,' said John, looking up at me through his thick pebble glasses. 'They've offered me a chance to be an air traffic controller. An air traffic controller!' he repeated bitterly. 'For God's sake, how could they let me go so far, knowing what was to come?'

I shook my head, having no answer. I still have none now.

The RAF, to my mind, had let him down in an appalling and unforgivable fashion.

Here was a young man whose whole life had until now been dedicated towards becoming a pilot, whose whole future had been built around acceptance into the service of his choice. And yet not one single person had pointed out to him that he was doomed to inevitable failure; not at the careers advisory office, nor his initial interview, and most heinous of all not at the moment he walked in through the door of Biggin Hill. It was almost criminal to let him undergo his eyesight test as the final investigation.

Well, John, wherever you may now be, I have no idea what happened to you after that day, or what career you subsequently took up. I would like to think that if you had stuck to your guns and approached some of the commercial airlines at least one of them might have taken a more sensible view. Whatever the case, I hope you somehow found a way to fulfil your dream, or at least as much of it as was humanly possible.

But the RAF and I?

Well, we hadn't exactly got off to the best of starts.

Several months after attending the session at Biggin Hill, it was time for the 'Big Challenge'.

All new RAF recruits – whatever their creed, colour or political persuasions – had to go undergo the IOT (Initial Officer Training) course at RAF Cranwell. This, I must explain, was intended to be a stamina-sapping process of undiluted purgatory, but they had reckoned without our formative training.

We were twenty-one doctors, a couple of dentists – and Bob, the token vicar, a bit like a token ethnic minority character in the early episodes of *Coronation Street*.

But Bob didn't see it quite that way, as we were later to find out.

There was, even with the benefit of hindsight, a distinct degree of friction between ourselves – mature, responsible members of society with our Greenpeace badges hidden surreptitiously behind our lapels – and them, the 'proper officers', ready to 'do or die' for their mother country. Although in 1983 there was precious little 'doing' that I was aware of, and without wishing to denigrate anyone who genuinely gave their life for our country, not a lot of dying either, especially for the greater cause of which we were all so desperate to become part.

The rivalry began from the start.

'Real' Air Force officers were subjected to a twelve-week induction course, whilst we doctors, dentists – and Bob – had to contend with a measly twenty-eight days of instruction.

'Real' Air Force men, sad deluded individuals that they were, inexplicably believed we were comparative lightweights, incapable of coping with twelve weeks of the worst that could be thrown at us. We doctors, dentists and Bob, however, uniformly modest to a fault, were at frequent pains to point out to them the collective error of their ways.

We, contrary to the universally accepted opinion, were under no such illusions. We were just so brimful of professional proficiency that we were indisputably capable of absorbing in just the one month of our comparatively laid-back training each and every relevant fact that they were in need of the full three for. And, more importantly, we were not required to get our hair cut so short, no matter how much the Sergeant Major barked at us.

We were doctors, and dentists and Bob, were we not? We were privileged.

But the truth is, on reflection, that we were older – older, but not necessarily more mature – and wiser, having been forged in the rigorous foundry of junior hospital jobs, an obligatory hell on earth. We were also supremely accustomed to the rigours of chronic sleep deprivation, having undergone the equivalent of advanced SAS training in that respect. Young doctors these days are rarely subjected to such mind-numbingly draining regimes, and this has a strange mixture of beneficial and deleterious consequences.

They have a life, for a start, and no longer walk around like the sedated zombie lookalikes we used to be. But at the same time – and unexpected though it may be, this is a serious observation – neither do they learn to practise medicine at the edge: at the edge of their energy, at the limits of their resources and of their patience. When you still have nigh on another forty years of your career to go, it can be – and was – a valuable lesson to be learned.

If you can survive house jobs you can survive anything.

So what was it like?

I give you three examples, none of which I pretend to be totally unique to me – others may have suffered worse, or more often. I once worked from a Thursday morning to a Monday evening, non-stop, and without pause for a minute's sleep. In no way would I have been at my most alert and competent in the latter stages of this mammoth shift, but who ever told the patients? Surely they had an inalienable right to expect a moderately sharp and committed doctor to attend to their emergency admission, but in truth I was generally more interested in retiring to my bed – or in fact any bed, whether already occupied or not – than in responding appropriately to any of their potentially life-threatening diseases.

On another occasion, similar to that detailed in my first book, my now ex-mother-in-law came to stay for a week, sharing the small, two-bedroom hospital flat I then occupied. I collected her from the station one Wednesday, and returned her there the following Tuesday.

Luckily for at least one of us, we did not meet in between.

If I was not working, I was out for the count on the ward. If I wasn't asleep on the ward I would be quietly dozing in casualty, or grabbing a quick ten minutes in the mortuary. This was indubitably the quietest spot in every hospital I've ever worked in – save at three in the morning, when every moribund patient in the world seems to breathe their last.

It's an as yet undisclosed conspiracy of major proportions, with the express intention of disturbing the poor junior doctor at the most inauspicious moment possible – i.e. just when he had arrived at the all-night party in the nurses' home for the fifth and final time that evening where the only thing that was not free was . . . well, it is a long time ago, and I have happily long since forgotten.

Thirdly, as a very junior physician carefully negotiating a tortuous path through my second hospital post, the unthinkable happened. I was then working in the comparatively relaxed atmosphere of what was known as a 'one in three' – no, this did not mean that one doctor had only three patients to see at any one particular time, even though it often felt like it. The sad but unavoidable reality was that you worked two twelve-hour day shifts followed by a twenty-four-hour day and night stint, after which the rota repeated itself again, and again, and again until you lost all semblance of who and where you were, what you were doing and why you were doing it.

All was going comparatively well until the last of the six months in the post when one of my rota-sharing colleagues decided to get married, and was under the obviously mistaken apprehension that a honeymoon should be taken, and immediately. Even that would have been bearable under the circumstances – the resulting 'one in two' being barely acceptable for a limited period had the light at the end of the tunnel not proved to be an on-rushing train.

My one remaining junior succumbed alarmingly to a life-threatening case of chickenpox, being admitted to the intensive care unit over the weekend . . .

This was not, I have to say, an entirely wasted experience on his behalf as he at last understood what a ventilator was for, but the fallout was such that I worked and was on call for twenty-four hours a day, seven days a week for the subsequent month. By the end of this nightmarish spell whatever intellectual capacity I may once have had was left totally scrambled, never completely to return.

In many respects such experiences were the making of me, my fellow IOT doctors and, in their own way, the dentists (not forgetting Bob). We were ready for anything and everything the Air Force might wish to throw at us – tough, case-hardened, and mostly hungover as we were. What completely mystified us, however, was how we had been subversively coerced into a Victorian regime that required us to have our hair cut more than once every other year and be polite to people we had neither previously met nor harboured any particular wish to encounter ever again.

The general rule of thumb was to be subservient to anyone with a better shine on their shoes than ourselves, or more stripes on their shoulder.

RAF Cranwell was an intriguing place.

The buildings and grounds were undeniably impressive, even

to such cynics as ourselves, and small groups of new recruits marched smartly across endless courtyards in their immaculate uniforms with a pride and a vigour in their step that you could not fail to admire. But these were small groups of new recruits that did not include doctors and dentists, that is, or Bob . . .

What united us was an unfailing inability to conform to any of the rules that we were subjected to, and the RAF's complete lack of comprehension as to why we could not. There was a devastatingly simple explanation for this.

We were mostly too worldly wise, too experienced in life on the outside – and let's face it, too damned recalcitrant – to be capable of conforming to anything. Anything at all.

And there were so many rules and regulations to abide by . . .

Among the twenty-three or so doctors and dentists – and Bob – there were, I think, some fourteen able-bodied men, a description to which Bob, for all his other undoubted attributes, would I am sure have never laid claim. There were also half a dozen or so able-bodied women, I hasten to add, a mixture of physiotherapists and nurses, but in light of what was to follow I plead complete absolution from any resultant form of sexual discrimination.

From memory, the 'real' officers on the course numbered approximately ninety-two, a small disparity of around seventy personnel in their favour. On the second night of our stay they challenged us to an inter-course hockey match.

We counted up those amongst our number who had played the game before and came up with the grand total of three – one of whom was myself, whose sole claim to fame was once to come on as an unexpected substitute late in the second half of a 'friendly' mixed hockey match in my fourth term at medical school. I still bear the scars.

We politely declined the offer.

They challenged us to a game of soccer instead, and smirking quietly, we accepted.

Of the fourteen aforementioned able-bodied men available to us, at least eight had played soccer before. Two of the rest were sufficiently large and ugly enough to be trained in the short term to kick anything wearing an opposition shirt anywhere that might make them squeal, and amongst the remaining four we found and unleashed our secret weapon.

Roger Hackney – and for once I have not changed a name – was then an Olympic 400 metres hurdles runner, and could run and run all day. True, neither he nor ourselves always knew where exactly he was running to, but as the game progressed into its latter stages we would just give him the ball and a compass and point to the opposition goal line shouting, 'That way.'

And that way he would go, trailing any number of 'real' officers in his wake.

Outnumbered, outsupported, but never outmanoeuvred or outplayed, we won deservedly 3–1. They never forgave us, particularly after the ensuing night of bar-games when we trounced them soundly at anything they cared to name.

At midnight that evening the entire complement of doctors, dentists – and Bob – raised our replenished glasses to the vanquished foe. There was not a single one of them to be seen.

The oppressive rules and regulations of the place were predeterminably doomed to start intruding into our lives, and it was of no surprise to anyone that we rapidly came to hate them unequivocally. It began with the obligatory haircuts, progressed rapidly to the trials and tribulations of the boot room and culminated in the endlessly tiresome task of saluting every senior officer you might encounter, whether in uniform or not.

'If it moves,' went the mantra of the day, 'salute it . . .'

This, I should point out, was Her Majesty's Forces' sense of humour at its finest.

' . . . and if it doesn't, paint it white.'

We tried, when and where we could, to obey all that we were

instructed to, but we were doctors, and dentists, and Bob – and mostly we failed. There was however one completely un-enforceable rule, one that we made not the least attempt to comply with. One, in fact, that we went as far out of our way as possible to break whenever and wherever we could.

The curfew . . .

At the time of writing Jack Straw, the present Home Secretary, has recently suggested imposing a curfew upon children. I forget the precise details – probably because he didn't really go into any – but the gist of it as far as I can recall was that juveniles under a certain age would, if found on the streets unaccompanied by an adult after a designated time, be forcibly rounded up by the police and returned home. This idea was swiftly abandoned, I believe, as being unworkable, most of our police force being safely tucked up in their beds long before the said little varmints emerge blinking into the light from the amusement arcades and opium dens they frequent.

As anyone with the merest hint of common sense will instantly realize, if it won't work with young children, it sure as hell won't work with grown-ups – like doctors, dentists and Bob.

We are just proud to be different.

And I'm sorry, but telling a twenty-five-year-old doctor – who is more than accustomed to working twenty-four and forty-eight-hour shifts without sleep – that he must be indoors by, say, 10.30 in the evening, and snuggled down soundly asleep by eleven . . . I ask you.

You might as well ask sheep to be intelligent.

Looking at it dispassionately, if you were to dictate to any group of doctors, dentists or Bobs that they were to be in bed by a given time on a given day, you would have about a one in ten chance of success. Or to put it in other words, if you were to direct ten doctors at any stage in their arrested development to be in bed at a certain hour, maybe one of them would actually achieve it – provided you did not state precisely whose bed he should be in, or how long he should stay there.

The RAF Cranwell approach to the matter – and our response – was equally simple and direct. They demanded that we should be back in the officers' quarters by eleven o'clock without fail, and locked every door and window in the county bang at the requisite hour to ensure our uninhibited compliance, and we . . .

Well, we took pride in paying no attention to this draconian directive at all.

It was a matter of principle. If we were given an order of which we did not approve, we would reserve our right to disobey it on any grounds we could think of. Had the currently much loved European Court of Human Rights then existed we would have been quoting it, loudly and often.

So the reality was that whilst all the 'proper' officer trainees – the poor lambs – were somnolently recumbent in their beds before 9 p.m., exhausted after a full day's travail and with their comforters still waiting expectantly to be unwrapped from their anonymized brown paper bags, we doctors, dentists and Bob were busy enjoying ourselves at as many far- flung places as you can envisage.

We had all learned the hard way how to live without sleep, and once no longer working we just wanted to have a little fun. Which we did, and were very nearly to pay the ultimate price for.

But Cranwell was more than just institutionalized boredom and a collection of outdated rules and regulations. There was a whole Bibleful of protocol to absorb, into the bargain.

When we arrived there, for example, we were immediately informed of the presence of the 'Royal Personage'. My first thought was that he would mumble a few incomprehensible words to us as a captive audience and be whisked away by lunchtime, but no. He was apparently here to stay.

After an overtly obsequious eulogy from the deputy Station Commander as to his finer points – an example of which we were to be intriguingly exposed to later – we were then subjected to an incomprehensively intricate explanation of how we were to greet him during a chance encounter in the 'corridors of power'. The details have long since been erased from my memory with the passing of the years – as, I suspect, have his temporary digestive problems to him – but it seemed to us all at the time to be impossibly complicated.

Upon our first meeting, as I recall, we were to call him 'Your Majesty'. Each subsequent meeting required a different form of address. He, on the other hand, could call us anything he wanted, but as he was an inoffensive sort of chap we anticipated that he would do no more than acknowledge our passing by inoffensively handing over his shoes, politely requiring us to polish them within the next twenty-four hours before returning them to his batman. A week into our stay we fully expected to be ironing his underwear, possibly with him still in it, but it wasn't like that at all.

By a process of extrapolation I duly calculated that come the seventh or eighth meeting we would just give him a high five, exclaim *Eastenders* style, 'Orl righ', mate?' and offer him a cigarette.

When it actually came to it, however, what would invariably happen was as follows. Generally there would be two or three of us wandering aimlessly together down the corridor, each of us having met him a different number of times, and there he would suddenly be, heading towards us. We would then metaphysically resort to scratching our heads, wondering what today's greeting should be, and mostly failing to come up with an answer.

At this point he would grin affably across, raise a casual hand in greeting and say good-humouredly before we had come to any significant conclusions, 'Hiyah, guys,' before ambling on.

From what limited exposure we had to him he did seem to be a thoroughly nice young man, although he often looked as if he yearned for some genuine company rather than living the enforced solitary existence foisted upon him by his unavoidable position in life's predetermined hierarchy. Effectively he was surrounded by people his own age who were wholly unable to approach him, and as we sat boisterously enjoying afternoon tea and toast in our ante-room we could often see him staring wistfully through the glass of the intervening door as he sat alone, with no one to talk to.

He did, however – lucky chap that he was – come complete with a bodyguard, who by popular consensus based on close observation appeared to have only two main pastimes in life. Number one – and these are not in any order of preference – drinking heavily, and to excess, from whatever moment the Cranwell bar opened each evening until whatever moment it closed. And number two, chatting up every available (but unaccountably unresponsive) female in sight.

Night after night he would roll out of the bar and off to his nocturnal duties more than a little the worse for wear. Night after night we too would roll out, rarely less than a couple of hours later, but there seemed to us a subtle though clearly definable difference. Whilst we might have a sneaking sense of sympathy for the Royal Personage, we were not actually being paid to protect him.

Come to think of it, we were not being paid at all. For anything.

Of course it had to happen, sooner or later.

After a particularly riotous evening towards the end of our induction period, a group of us returned to Cranwell from the local den of iniquity masquerading as a 'Typical English Pub'. We were, strangely, only marginally the worse for wear and more than prepared for the early morning ritual of avoiding the guards and breaking back into the officers' quarters. The general plan was for one of our number – preferably inhabiting a room on the ground floor – to leave a window slightly ajar through which we would all quietly file (well, as quietly as half a dozen solemnly inebriated physicians could manage) before dispersing to our own beds.

On this particular night the unfortunate person with whom the responsibility lay – OK, it was me – had forgotten to leave his window open, making re-entry a bit of a problem. As we had already acquired the second of our official warnings for being caught out of bounds, this presented something of a dilemma. There was no alternative. After tiptoeing stealthily around the perimeter of the building, looking for any available point of access, to our great relief we eventually stumbled across an open window.

We stopped outside and listened. All seemed peaceful within. One by one we crept in, exhorting each other in stage whispers to absolute silence.

'No giggling,' I can recall somebody saying. 'And no breaking of wind.'

Six people immediately started laughing. As they stopped, a distant and undisclosed seventh announced his alimentary disinhibitions with some ferocity . . .

We drew together in a tight-knit group in the centre of the room, enveloped by the complete darkness as we held our breaths, wondering where the door and our subsequent point of egress should be. But we need not have worried, as it suddenly found us.

The door burst open, the light flooded on, and there – flamboyantly attired in surprisingly well-tailored tartan pyjamas – stood the royal bodyguard. Gun in hand, legs astride and his voice thick with alcohol he exuded more menace than I would have ever thought him capable.

'Halt!' he shouted. (I thought this only happened in films.) 'Who goes there?'

As our eyes slowly adjusted to the light we looked around us to see where on earth we had landed. To one side of the room we realized there was a bed, and in that bed a body. It was a hot night, and the body had evidently felt in no need of pyjamas. It looked rather familiar, in a strange sort of way.

The body moved, and raised a hand.

'Hiyah, guys,' said our royal friend, grinning from ear to ear.

The last lecture was over, the last seminar complete and the last lesson learned – after a fashion. All that remained to transform us from fledgling Flying Officer cadets into fully trained, supremely fit, state of the art fighting machines . . . oh, all right, to marginally more qualified doctors, dentists and Bob . . . was our passing out parade the following morning.

But it wasn't as simple as it might have sounded.

We had to march past the Station Commander in perfect drill order, saluting smartly, undertake a few adroit left and right turns and finish off in style with the odd twiddly manoeuvre encompassing sufficient panache and expertise to meet his critical approval.

'Piece of cake,' we reassured each other slightly uneasily. 'Should be a doddle.'

But training wasn't going all that well.

'You're not even as good as bloody useless,' bellowed the long-suffering Warrant Officer Williams, our hapless trainer, frustratedly after our final training session the afternoon before our big day. 'In fact – begging your pardons, madams and sirs – accusing you of incompetence on a grand scale combined with complete lack of effort or application would be an understatement comparable to saying the Grand Canyon is quite a nice hole in the ground. I know you're only doctors and dentists . . . '

'And Bob,' someone reminded him.

' . . . and Bob,' he acknowledged with a reluctant grin, 'but I've had doctors, dentists and Bobs before during my untold years in Her Majesty's Forces, and they have always been at least encroaching upon the unacceptably abject, but you lot

. . . You are my last cohort, I'm due to retire at the weekend, and I had always wanted to go out on a high, proud of all I had achieved . . . '

Words seemed to fail him as he threw his arms helplessly in the air.

' . . . words fail me,' he continued, without appearing to draw breath. 'I am fully aware that none of you rabidly ineffectual shower intend to pursue a career as parade ground officers, but where is your self-respect, for goodness sake? You just don't seem to care. Have you no pride in yourselves, no wish to present yourselves in the best light, however dim that may be? I've seen more illumination in the Black Hole of Calcutta. But it's not just me you're letting down; it's yourselves, and more importantly all the legions of colleagues who came before you, and will come after.'

He shrugged his shoulders and made to walk away, before pausing and turning back.

'I like you lot,' he added exasperatedly. 'I don't know why, but I've actually enjoyed working with you, after a fashion. I don't want to end my career being so disappointed in you all.'

'Looks good for tomorrow, then,' I observed optimistically as we filed thoughtfully off the square.

'Shut up, Mike,' chorused everyone within earshot.

We sat discussing the situation over dinner that night.

'So what's it to be?' asked Tim, one of the two dentists on the course. 'An extra training session this evening, or . . . ?'

He glanced around at our assembled group, all of us shaking our heads dolefully.

'Then a pub crawl it is,' he announced decisively. 'Any absentees . . . no, Lawrence, I wasn't actually including you amongst the ranks of those whose opinions we seek,' as the aforementioned Lawrence raised his hand tentatively. 'Anyone else with a degree of credibility? Good. I suggest we all meet in the foyer at eight.'

With dinner, as it was our last night, came wine, and plenty of it, so there was a slight but understandable delay. By 8.45, however, we were duly assembled as directed, boldly to venture forth in search of adventure, excitement, and entertainment . . . yes, even within the regional environs of Cranwell. And happily we found it, returning through the station grounds in the early hours of the morning in time-honoured fashion, re-entering via the tried and trusted open window technique – only one of ours, this time.

A little judicious forethought now reaped its reward. The bar, as we fully anticipated, had long since closed, but we turned in the opposite direction, filing silently through the deserted corridors to arrive in the oppressive darkness at our intended destination, a small, mostly unused ante-room towards the rear of the building. We switched on the lights and there we were, ready to carry on where we had left off in our impromptu 'Blue Peter' bar – as in 'Here's one I prepared earlier . . . '

By four in the morning even we were fading.

'Got to march tomorrow,' Nigel, a broadly built Northerner reminded us, 'and I believe we are officially crap. "Worst I've ever seen," didn't WO Williams say – or words to that effect?'

'Well, that's something to be proud of, isn't it?' I suggested brightly. ' . . . I guess perhaps it isn't,' I finished lamely, ducking the variety of inanimate objects suddenly heading my way.

'*No!*' expostulated Bob suddenly, crashing his fist down on the table in a most unreverential fashion and making us jump almost as much as the glasses still upon it. 'No, no, no, no, no! This will not do.'

'There's a worryingly evangelical glint in your eye,' I said. 'Sort of frightening.'

'Good,' he responded forcefully, 'because I'm a vicar and evangelical glinting is what I'm supposed to be best at. Look, it gets light at five o'clock, this time of year. What do you say – let's grab an hour and a half's sleep and meet on the parade ground at 6.30. An hour's practice before breakfast – who knows what we might manage.'

'No,' responded one and all unanimously. 'Absolutely no. Not a chance of it.'

'God would be proud of you,' said Bob enticingly . . .

At 6.30 on the dot we assembled in the parade ground, every man Jack and Jill of us, and began marching in the early morning light as if our lives depended upon it. A totally trans-formed Bob was our driving force, our inspiration, revealing a hitherto unsuspected Sergeant Majorish ferocity, an impressively stentorian voice and a whole new earthy range of vocabulary – not to mention an unexpectedly nifty pair of feet.

At 7.30 we broke for breakfast, and by eight o'clock we were out on the square again, under Bob's hawk-like eye, fully equipped with our incontinence devices. And by 8.30 . . .

'Got it,' breathed Bob triumphantly. 'I do believe we've got it . . .'

The passing out parade was traditionally followed by a grand ceremonial dinner. It was a 'more than three knives' affair in the intimidating presence of the Station Commander and other noble dignitaries, to mark our initiation into the ranks, an event we had all been secretly dreading. But now . . .

Loath that we would ever have been to admit it, we were rather proud of ourselves, we doctors, dentists and Bob. Four weeks earlier we had begun our time at Cranwell as an unruly, ill-disciplined rabble, only to go rapidly downhill from there. When we left to depart in our ultimately disparate directions we would no doubt swiftly return to type, but for one short spell, for one never to be forgotten moment, we had marched, turned, saluted and stood rigidly to attention as if to the manner born.

It was beyond our wildest dreams.

'I'm proud of you, madams and sirs,' said Warrant Officer

Williams, who had been watching the event with a bemused expression on his face. 'Bloody amazed, if you'll excuse me saying so, but proud of you all the same. It was the best I've ever seen.'

5

Little Men with Big Egos – and Vice Versa

After a short break – to consult a marriage guidance counsellor – it was off from Cranwell to RAF Chivenor, just outside Barnstaple in North Devon.

My first posting, and the excitement was . . . underwhelming.

I drove down there the weekend before I was due to start and found most of my future colleagues enjoying themselves at a barbecue in the medical centre grounds, spit-roasting an administrative sergeant. The Senior Medical Officer – henceforth referred to as the SMO, the Air Force being awash with abbreviations – who was to be my immediate boss for the next eighteen months, proved to be an amiable chap in his early thirties, already weighed down with the responsibility of three young children.

I was then approaching the tender age of twenty-five, and still openly ageist. 'My God,' was my immediate thought upon our first meeting. 'How grown up, how very middle-aged. How boring.'

I am now forty-six, with four children of my own. How times change.

RAF Chivenor, although the home of the wonderfully efficient Search and Rescue (SAR) helicopter squadron, was primarily a training base for fast jet pilots – 'La crème de la crème', as they liked to call themselves. If the young students were to pass successfully through here – and by no means all of them did,

104

especially if I had my way – they would have finally made it on to the big stage, the realization of their dream.

Much to my surprise, I quickly learned that crashing a plane and disposing of a few million pounds of the Armed Forces' resources appeared to be by no means an insuperable obstacle to success. There was, indeed, a certain amount of awe surrounding the select band of pilots who had ejected in full flight and lived to survive the tale – even more so had they sustained the ultimate badge of honour, the odd crushed vertebra or two.

This was a club whose membership I was keen to avoid.

Several jets vanished into the deep pockets of the tax-paying public during my tenure, most spectacularly in the course of a mid-air collision over the sea, in which thankfully no one was injured. More entertaining, however – from a strictly uninvolved bystander's point of view – was the jet which dropped like the proverbial stone from the sky during a late night training session in early autumn. Unencumbered by the usual protocol it slithered to a halt – metal screeching and sparks flying – less than a hundred yards from the officers' mess, where a group of us were enjoying an after-dinner drink . . . though come to think of it, dinner had finished three or four hours earlier.

The emergency alarm sounded soon afterwards, which in time-honoured tradition everyone present first ignored.

'These bloody training exercises,' said an older, more experienced and greater girthed officer to my left. 'I wish they wouldn't –'

We were never to know what he wished they wouldn't, because the alarm sounded again almost immediately, but a little more loudly this time. And in case any of us had missed the extreme seriousness of the situation a voice intoned solemnly over the Tannoy system, 'We have a plane down. We have a plane down to the north-east of the runway . . . '

'Where's that?' I asked, interested.

'About . . . there,' said the man to my left, pointing just outside the window.

'All personnel are to evacuate the building immediately,' continued the announcer in rising hysteria. 'There is a clear and immediate fire risk to . . . '

I shall never know quite what to, despite the fact that a junior officer at the other end of the bar, somewhat the worse for wear, shouted out, 'His trousers . . . ' before ducking for cover. Meanwhile I was diverted by that intriguing phenomenon, my first experience of witnessing servicemen responding to a major event without quite knowing what they were supposed to be doing. To summarize as best I can, I would say that everyone found an obviously predesignated collection of small circles in which to run around for an equally predetermined length of time before congregating in a curious array of designer all-weather gear on the edge of the runway, a matter of yards from the smoking wreckage of the crashed jet. Of the pilot there was no sign.

'Do the fuel tanks never explode then?' I asked innocently, seeing a look of horror sink into the face of the young officer standing next to me. 'And, given the fact that the pilot is obviously somewhere other than where we all are, and that most of the plane would appear to be unlikely to be getting airborne again in the immediate future — unless something in it were to detonate within the next few minutes — what the bloody hell are we doing here?'

'Good point,' he said thoughtfully, walking steadily backwards away from me before being swallowed up by the surrounding darkness.

'We must organize a search party,' somebody called out urgently.

What for? I wanted to reply, though thankfully for my immediate safety keeping my mouth shut. 'The plane's just over there, look, that twisted grey metal thing with flames spurting out of the tail section . . . '

The search party was not an unqualified success, primarily because it was pitch black and none of them could see each other, not to mention the fact that nobody had the least idea in which direction to start searching. The circles they were running in became ever smaller, and more tightly knit.

And my part in this disorganized debacle? Well, I was the new boy, standing quietly to one side, trying not to get in the way and watching with some interest as the SAR helicopter sped unnoticed at low altitude round the airfield perimeter to collect the pilot from where he lay bobbing gently in the river, having located his rescue beacon from the control tower.

My introduction to the world of RAF station life was interesting – not necessarily pleasurable, but educational nonetheless.

The hierarchical structure took a little getting used to. As a house officer, the most junior of the doctors in the NHS, there had been above me a senior house officer (SHO), above him a junior registrar, a senior registrar, and bestriding the world like a Colossus, the consultant. We respected them for their professional prowess; they were more experienced than us, had more letters after their name, and rarely had to sleep fully dressed in the sluice room.

Doctors in charge of doctors – that I could cope with. But in the RAF . . .

I was still only a year after qualification, and had much to learn from my superiors, who were . . . above me, Reg, the SMO, for whom I had the greatest respect. And above him . . . Wing Commander Short, an apt name which could have been apter had he borne the far more appropriate soubriquet of Wing Commander Short, Fat and Officially Obnoxious.

Because Wing Commander SFOO was not a doctor at all, but an administrator with an ego and self-importance as large as his stature was insufficient.

We did not get off to the best of starts.

I eventually spent six years in the RAF, for my sins, and for most of that time I was pretty much a marked man. I was generally one of only two or three doctors on the camp, drove a car with 'Doctor' emblazoned across the side of it (bit of a give-away, really) and had my very own green flashing light. Then there was this unerring habit of rubbing people up the wrong way. That is, the entire Air Force had this habit, and doctors were generally the people being the wrong way rubbed.

To get to the medical centre at Chivenor you passed through the main gates separating the camp from the married quarters and it was less than fifty yards ahead on the left. When I arrived to take up my post of JMO — Junior Medical Officer — the entrance was being renovated and the building works were such that the area was impassable. They were enlarging the guard house to accommodate the jacuzzi and a new rest room where the guards could recover from their arduous duties — pressing one button to raise the gate, for example, and a completely different one to lower it — by watching pornographic videos and playing Russian roulette with the station cat.

The net result of this was that you had to drive three and a half miles round the perimeter of the airfield to reach the medical centre, which instead of being the first building you encountered on arrival was now the last. In an emergency, doctors and rescue squads could drive across the airfield at a set point, although the only time I attempted to do this myself it wasn't actually an emergency, and I did not quite manage to cross at the appropriate set point.

Should you be wondering how this happened, bear in mind it was dark (which it usually is at 2.30 in the morning), the sailing club bar had been open an awfully long time, and draw your own conclusions. Still, no real harm was done — save for the irreversible destruction of the automatic bird scarer and I did manage to retrieve the car at first light the next morning.

There was a strict speed limit of 40 mph on the perimeter track, but generally very little traffic in evidence at any one time. A long clear road, a ridiculous speed limit, and the fact that I was driving somebody else's car — well, what would you have done?

So it was purely by good luck that just as I was entering my own personal speeding zone I happened to spot in the rear-view mirror the car belonging to Wing Commander Short following behind me.

I drove impeccably. Even I was surprised.

The journey being completed without event, I pulled up at the medical centre some thirty seconds after the Wing Commander had arrived at Station Headquarters. As I strolled into Reg's office to say 'Good morning' I found him on the phone. He covered the mouthpiece with one hand and motioned me to sit down.

'It's Wing Commander "Admin",' he mouthed. 'He's just telling me how he followed you round the perimeter track.'

I sat down. Nice of the Wing Commander to ring and congratulate me on the quality of my driving, I thought, feeling an unaccustomed warm glow towards him in particular, and for the first time in my life just about any administrator anywhere.

'Yes, sir,' said Reg, wincing slightly as he continued his conversation. 'He's just come in.' There was a moment's silence, and then he looked at me, completely deadpan.

'He says there's a 40 mph speed limit on the perimeter road,' he said, 'and for over half a minute or so you were doing 42. He'd like to see you in his office.'

I know. It's hard to believe that people can be that petty, but the combination of administration and Wing Commandership is a pretty heady mix. We had many such interesting conversations in his office during the following eighteen months, and I generally felt I had the moral victory. Unfortunately for me, however, the Wing Commander had the greater rank, and victories had to be a great deal more than moral to counter this tiny disadvantage.

But I got my own back, in the end. And best of all it was in a moment of pleasure all the more supreme because it was from a position of such apparent impotence . . .

They have a quaint custom in the Air Force, when a new officer arrives at a station, of 'dining him in' at the first mess night of his stay. A mess night is an obligatory jamboree where all the officers dress up like Savoy Hotel doormen and stay up drinking too late with a group of colleagues they have to try to pretend they like for as long as they can manage.

The Station Commander and the mess secretary then each make a speech, trying usually in vain to summon up one good joke between them. During the after-dinner cigars and passing of the port they move on to say how nice it is to welcome Flight Lieutenant so and so to his new post, how much they are looking forward to working with him and how lucky we all are to have him / her join our happy band. And yes, they even said that about me, if you were wondering.

This ritual is trotted out on a regular basis, on the strict understanding that when we eventually leave the station, and are subsequently 'dined out', we reciprocate by saying equally nice things about everyone we have been working with.

'It has been so nice to work with you,' we are supposed to intone. 'You are such a nice group of people. We have bonded so well, and I shall miss you all terribly. The future will be a bleaker place without you. Only grey days shall now follow . . . '

My dining out night duly arrived. I was the most junior of seven officers being dined out, and was therefore not expected to speak.

But I had already made my plans . . .

After pre-dinner drinks, we all filed dutifully into the dining room. The portents were not auspicious.

The top table beckoned, strung along one end of the room. I glanced at the seating plan and all but gave up. I was seated at the far left of the table, the end, the most isolated position of all. And who should be sitting next to me, cutting me off from all recognized forms of human contact? Wing Commander Short, of course.

I sat, and I ate, and I thought furiously. Common sense suggested that I swallow my pride, accept defeat, and disappear quietly into the distance. But that was common sense.

Dinner eaten, cigars smoked and speeches spoken, the dreaded moment arrived. The Station Commander – 'God With a Funny Hat' – duly introduced me.

'It is unusual,' he said, 'for us to dine out seven officers in the one evening. It is even more unusual that they should all turn up. But it is particularly unusual . . . ' and he paused for effect, because he was that sort of man, 'for the seventh, and by far the most junior, of our departees to not only wish to speak, but all but demand to do so. I give you – if you should want him – Flight Lieutenant Sparrow.'

He sat down to a rousing silence as the assembled pilots, administrators, engineers, honoured guests and all the serving staff (crowding in from the now empty kitchen) sat, or stood, and waited with a varying degree of bated breaths.

The floor was mine.

It is now nearly twenty years ago, and as I write I realize I have scarcely thought about that night since, yet I can recall every word, every phrase – though perhaps it were better that I should not.

I took a deep breath, and off I went. The Wing Commander – the only person I had hitherto been in a position to speak to throughout the evening – sat smugly beside me, polishing his balding head with a damp handkerchief. As I opened my mouth to speak he smiled patronizingly up at me, secure in the unshakeable sanctity of his exalted position.

So it wasn't my fault. It was that smile that did it.

'Station Commander, honoured guests, ladies and gentlemen,'

I began, 'and you lot over in the corner there,' pointing at the pilots.

Silence. Off to a good start, then. I ploughed on, regardless.

'When I arrived here this evening, like all of you, I went to look at the seating plan to see who I was lucky enough to be located next to. You can imagine my surprise – and you will have to imagine my delight – at finding I was sitting right at the end here, next to the Wing Commander.'

The entire room took a deep breath.

'I wondered why this was, ' I continued, entirely unabashed – it was far too late to be abashed now. 'Was it for the benefit of my company, perhaps? My witty repartee, my knowledge-able discourse upon the state of the nation, or merely a coincidence?'

I took a leaf out of the Station Commander's book, then, and paused for my own effect. They had been holding their breath for so long a lot of their faces were beginning to turn purple.

'As the evening wore on, and the main course was served, I realized it was none of these things,' and I paused again, but I think this time it was due more to abject panic.

'It was so I could cut up his food for him,' I finished simply.

Now, I've never actually heard a pin drop, or a fairy sneeze, but if ever there was a moment when you might, then this would have been it.

Complete, unmitigated, absolute . . . silence.

I waited, wondering idly if there was still time for a court martial before the evening was out. And then suddenly, wonderfully, somebody started chuckling, and then the whole place degenerated into gales of laughter.

I warmed to my theme.

'I was dined out by the administrative wing, last week, along with three of my fellow guests tonight. They gave us all £20 to buy something to remind us of RAF Chivenor. Flying Officer Parkwood bought a wall-mounted plaque, Flight Lieutenant

Thorpe some RAF cufflinks, and Flight Lieutenant Sheila Jenkins donated it to the RAF Benevolent Fund.'

Pause. I'm on a roll now.

'And me . . . ? I went to buy two hundred cigarettes and some dog food.'

I was starting to sweat, but there was more uproar, if anything.

'And then I reconsidered. I wanted to take with me something reminiscent of the department I have so joyously belonged to, a reminder of the boss who has done so . . . ' This would be a tear-welling-in-the-eye moment. ' . . . so little to further my career. So I bought this,' I added calmly.

I took possibly the deepest breath of my entire life and bent down to reach beneath my seat, where the mess manager had carefully hidden my prize possession when no one was watching. A garden gnome.

I held it aloft, and silence returned. There are times in your life when you can do no wrong, and this just seemed to be one of them. I let it roll.

'Now this is not just any old garden gnome,' I explained soberly. 'It's been specially adapted to fit a garden fountain. The water comes out here, look,' pointing to the relevant anatomical area, 'and I thought it to be the most appropriate memento possible because . . . ' Another pause, another collective intake of breath, another quick thought as to whether I would ever don a stupid uniform again ' . . . because it sits on its arse all day and pisses on everything underneath it.'

It was magical.

Even I, as I said it, murmured to myself, 'career-ending moment here, Mike,' but it was all too much for the assembled populace. They rose to a man – well, all but one – and a woman, and cheered, and applauded, and whooped with undisguised glee. I think, at this point, I should gloss over the rest of my speech – I would like to aim at a family audience – and merely bring you gently to the end.

'And finally a word to all you pilots out there. Some of you will be reaching puberty pretty soon ... ' I had to stop for a moment or two, until I could make myself heard again. ' ... and I have to tell you that this is a time of growth, of maturation, of assumption of responsibility. So perhaps, when this should happen, one of you could wander across to the administration department ... ' Final nail in the coffin here. ' ... and tell them what it is like.'

And with that I turned and walked out, cheers ringing in my ears. It was one of those moments you treasure for ever. Well, until the next day, that is.

The following morning found me in the Station Commander's office, standing to attention and wondering how a future in the refuse collection trade might be. He sat and regarded me in an almost paternal fashion, whilst I practised mental grovelling and abrogation.

'Nice speech, Mike,' he said thoughtfully. 'But I don't think you and the Air Force are destined to spend an awful lot of time together. Do you?'

After eighteen roller-coaster months at Chivenor it was finally onwards and upwards – geographically speaking – to RAF St Athan. This was large engineering station in South Wales, possibly the last place on earth a Celt-hating Mary's student would ever wish to be. To my great surprise, however, I discovered that some of the local inhabitants did have fully functional inside toilets after all.

I had, I soon discovered, been lucky with Reg as my first SMO. He had been ideal, the perfect combination of friend and gentle guiding hand through the as yet unknown intricacies of general practice. My new boss at St Athan – Donald – was an altogether different proposition. A small, dour, obsessional Scot, he had all the charisma of a house brick, but was of less practical use.

I was intrigued by the desk in his office, which was covered by a sheet of clear perspex under which he kept an array of charts, references and tables of normal medical values to refer to during consultations.

'It's ever so neat,' I said innocently to Simon, one of the young airmen working in the medical centre.

'He measures them,' he told me. 'Every night before he goes home. I saw him do it one day. Each one has to be so many inches from the side and the front first thing in the morning.'

'You're joking,' I said, disbelieving. 'No . . . ' I continued as he solemnly shook his head at me, 'you're not joking at all, are you?'

It was irresistible. Every now and then — not too often to be suspicious — Simon and I would sneak into his office after work and move all his little bits of paper, just a quarter of an inch or so, creeping out again like a naughty schoolboys, giggling helplessly.

Donald and I had many disagreements during my two and a half years there, but matters came to a head late one Monday afternoon after I had spent a long and for once arduous weekend on call. A non-urgent request for a visit had come in early that morning and Donald, being the duty doctor for the day, had been given the set of notes to deal with later, as was customary practice there.

'I'm off home now, Simon,' I said at around six o'clock, some five hours after I was due to have departed, 'for a well-deserved bath, a gut-buster of a gin and tonic and the biggest, fattest cigar South Wales has to offer. See you in the morning.'

'Um . . . sir . . . ' Simon was hovering uncertainly.

'Whatever it is, the answer is no,' I said emphatically. 'Even if it should be yes. I'm . . . OK, Simon, what is it?' I finished wearily, catching the wary look on his face. 'An emergency bunion in the waiting room? The Station Commander wants to invite me home for a sweet sherry? My wife has run off with the rag-and-bone man? What, Simon, what? I'm knackered, I want to go home, I want to . . . '

I drew to a halt.

'The boss wants you to do this visit before you go home,' he said, screwing his face up apologetically and holding the set of notes protectively in front of him in case I began spitting venom. 'Don't hit me, sir, or not with anything hard and pointed. I did try to tell him . . . '

'It's the visit that came in this morning, isn't it?' I snapped. 'Sorry, Simon,' relenting immediately, 'I know it's not your fault. But it is, isn't it?'

'It . . . sort of is, sir, yes,' he admitted. 'Would you . . . ? Do you mind . . . ? It might be advisable, under the circumstances.'

I rubbed my chin, and considered. 'Simon,' I said at last, 'have you ever seen a grown man cry?'

'Not recently, sir.'

'Then best you go home,' I suggested. 'Do you have anything else left to do?'

'Apparently not,' he said, gathering up his bags hurriedly. 'But sir . . . '

'Yesss,' I hissed.

'Please don't do anything we might any of us regret in the morning. Please . . . ?'

The building was empty, save for Donald and myself. I collected my thoughts, took a deep breath and knocked at the door of his consulting room.

'Yes?' he acknowledged grudgingly as I walked in.

'This,' I said evenly, glancing down at the set of notes in my hand, 'is the visit that came in this morning. Your visit. And this . . . ' hurling them forcibly against the wall and watching with dispassionate interest as the inners cascaded all over his meticulously organized desk, 'is an expression of my discontent at being asked to do it at the end of what was supposed to be my afternoon off.'

Donald's face was visibly paling.

'I am not,' I continued, with what I still like to think was a steely expression in my eyes, 'however you might regard me, some sort of subservient underling to whom you can delegate your unwanted business. And I am not,' digging my fingers into the palms of my hands to save me from wrapping them round his neck, 'taking any more of the derogatory crap that you have been throwing at me for the past couple of years. But most of all . . .'

I stopped in mid-flight, narrowing my eyes as he cowered back into his chair. The floor was mine.

' . . . I am not, repeat *not*, doing this sodding visit. You are.'

He rallied for a moment, sitting up in his seat and looking frantically for a finger to wag.

'I think you have forgotten something,' he began, gaining confidence. 'I am in charge here, and you are . . .'

He ground to a halt, that steely-eyed stuff no doubt taking effect.

'The doors are closed,' I informed him quietly. 'Everyone else has gone home. There's only you and me left. Within these four walls . . .'

It was awful. I felt an attack of the giggles coming on as I had a sudden vision of the unsung Googie Withers as a prison governor in the cult *Within These Walls* ITV drama in the late seventies. I wanted to ask him how he disposed of his greying nasal hair.

' . . . within these four walls,' I repeated, gathering myself just in time, 'there is no one, save you and I. No one to hear us, no one to judge, no one to pull me up for the undoubted insubordination I am about to display, and no one to come down on you like a ton of bricks for failing to fulfil your professional duty. This . . .' pointing to the set of notes still partially adhering to the wall, '

. . . is your visit, not mine. This . . . ' lifting up his medical bag and dumping it on the desk, ' . . . is a piece of equipment you might like to take with you. And this . . . ' leaning forward and glowering at him across his beautifully arranged perspex table top, ' . . . is a Flight Lieutenant who is no longer going to cover your arse purely because I need your signature on a piece of paper to verify I have completed the first part of my general practice training. Over to you. Oh, sorry sir, in my haste and utmost displeasure I had completely forgotten you were a senior officer, but now I remember . . . I don't care, and I'm going home.'

Life was never quite the same again, after that.

Although based at one station we were often sent to another to cover a colleague's sick leave, for example, or holidays, and it was for this reason I found myself working for a short spell at a base somewhere near Reading. For reasons that have long since escaped my memory, however, instead of returning to St Athan I was from there sent on a two-week course to RAF Halton, somewhere near Aylesbury.

A simple enough task to arrive there, you might think, save for the fact that I was at the time temporarily without a car, had very little sense of direction, and needed to negotiate the public transport system via Paddington en route. The same Paddington, I should point out, where St Mary's Hospital Medical School – that kindergarten for the under-privileged where I had spent five years thinking up excuses for my inability to attend lectures before lunchtime (and, if I'm totally honest, afterwards as well) – still resided, as did some half a dozen public houses I had spent so much of my formative years in.

I slipped into one of them for a restorative quick pint and a little self-indulgent reminiscence, and staggered out of another of them several hours and three phone calls to Halton later. I caught the last train – just – from Marylebone (I think), dis-embarked at the correct station by some miracle or other, and in the complete absence of any taxis walked the two and a half miles to the camp, carrying my bags. For some unaccountable reason, there was no one there to greet me.

I had, however, had the foresight to ask someone in the officers' mess to leave a door open and unlocked for me . . . and it may be that he did, but he failed to specify which one, and I was unable to precisely locate it. Undeterred – being locked out of where I was supposed to be, seriously inebriated at 2.30 in the morning, was a situation I was not entirely unaccustomed to – I found an open-ground floor window, threw in my suitcase, threw in my RAF officer's cap and then, in a resounding finale, threw in myself.

I am uncertain about the precise landing arrangements of my suitcase or my cap, but I at least had an enjoyably soft landing – on the rather large abdomen of the heavily slumbering figure on the bed just beneath the window. To my continuing amazement he just grunted, turned noisily over and went back to sleep. I thanked God silently, retrieved my cap and my suitcase after a few moments' fumbling in the dark and fled up the nearest staircase to bed.

There was just one small problem.

I did not know where my bedroom was, and so I improvised – in other words, I opened every door I came across until I found an unoccupied bed, having first found rather a lot of full ones. I emerged from the depths of unconsciousness the next morning secure in the knowledge that I had successfully negotiated the first hurdle of my stay with an undoubted degree of aplomb, but with just a hint of that vaguely uneasy feeling you have when the night before is a memory you have yet to make a complete and unexpurgated reacquaintance with.

That vaguely uneasy feeling ceased to be vague at all when I opened my eyes and saw the cap on the floor beside me. Something mysterious had happened to it overnight. Someone had obviously sneaked in under cover of darkness and sewn huge amounts of yellow braiding on to it (scrambled egg, as it was colloquially known).

I picked it up tremulously, and peered inside the rim.

Strange things do sometimes happen in this weird and wonderful world of ours, but being promoted five whole ranks above your former station whilst asleep in a strange mess, without your express permission, and having your surname changed into the bargain is not generally one of them.

'Air Commodore Stourscombe,' I read on the label.

'How the . . . ?' I began to wonder, and then with a sense of deeply impending doom I suddenly realized exactly how the . . . after all. It looked as if my stay was destined to be one of those short but interesting ones that generally ended up with an in-depth interview in front of a distinctly unamused high-ranking senior officer. There was only one thing to do. Lie unashamedly.

I dressed, and went down to breakfast.

Slowly, the dining room cleared, and just two late breakfasters remained. The other, a vast giant of a man in his middle fifties, glanced across at me from the end of the table, a benign smile – at least I hoped fervently it was a smile – playing at the corner of his lips. He was watching me, I noticed, and my heart began to sink.

After a few minutes more of observation he rose from his chair with surprising ease for a man of his bulk, walked across to where I was struggling unequally with the top of the Marmite pot, and sat down beside me.

'I guess that you're not actually Air Commodore Stourscombe,' he said after a short pause, regarding me thoughtfully.

I swallowed hard. 'No, sir,' I admitted, somewhat unnecessarily. 'I guess not.'

He nodded imperceptibly. 'Thought so,' he said evenly. 'And therefore I don't suppose I can be Flight Lieutenant Sparrow, can I?'

I swallowed harder. 'I don't suppose you can, sir,' I agreed.

'But if it helps at all, right at this moment, I don't think that you would actually want to be.'

The twitching at the corner of his mouth broadened into a full-blown smile. 'That will be of some comfort to my wife,' he said, stroking his upper lip.

I abandoned the thankless struggle with the lid of the Marmite jar with a sigh and, putting it down, looked up at him in complete submission. My fate was in his hands.

'They warned me about you,' he continued, biting his upper lip as if trying to prevent a belly laugh from breaking out, 'but I didn't expect quite such an explosive introduction. Please, Flight Lieutenant Sparrow . . . may I have my cap back?'

He was a big man, the Air Commodore, in more ways than one. If only the Air Force had had a few more like him.

Back at St Athan, a year or so after my ignominious encounter with Air Commodore Stourscombe, I was now well into the third of the six or so long years for which I graciously bestowed the dubious benefit of my company upon the RAF. Unaccountably I had found myself amongst an assembled array of luminous dignitaries gathered together in the officers' mess. We were watching a concert given with extreme professionalism by the RAF military band.

This, I have to say, was made all the more impressive by the fact that although we reposed snugly in the warm, dry confines of the mess entrance hall, they were standing outside in the cold, the dark and the pouring rain, less than a dozen yards in front of us.

Unfortunately I had arrived amidst said dignitaries – numbering senior officers and their wives, local eminencies with their worthy and aged relations and other 'Upstanding People of Import' from the community together with what they pretended to the rest of us were their 'families' – via the officers' mess bar. Instead, therefore, of standing smartly to attention and in reverential silence I had sadly given what I thought to be a witty, urbane and sotto voce running commentary throughout the entire proceedings.

As the band played their final rousing chorus before scampering off to some well-deserved shelter and a cup of hot chocolate, and as the gathering of the great and the good turned back to file thankfully into the warmth of the mess for the official post-concert reception, a loud voice bellowed out across the airwaves.

'Flight Lieutenant Sparrow. I want a word with you.'

'You can hear him,' murmured a fellow junior officer in my ear, 'but see him can you not.'

The assembled company parted obligingly, revealing the smallest officer on the station – Wing Commander Colclough – who had just a moment previously been obscured in their midst. Small in the physical stature department, he was unquestionably large in the 'I have an ego to be reckoned with' stakes and this was obviously a moment when he felt it pertinent to demonstrate his capabilities to the full.

Everyone present fell silent, weighing up the odds with some amusement. They might not have formerly considered it money well spent to witness a senior officer cut down a junior one to his appropriate size, but this was for free, and in no way were they inclined to miss out on the ensuing entertainment.

'I heard you, Flight Lieutenant Sparrow, make no mistake about it,' hissed the Wing Commander ominously, pointing out towards the terrace. 'And a thoroughly disgraceful display it was too,' he continued – which of course was completely true. It had to be deserving of virtually any sort of chastisement he wished to dispense in my general direction. But . . .

One of the golden rules of the RAF was that senior officers should never, under any circumstances, tear strips off their juniors in front of other ranks, and absolutely never, *ever* indulge in the same behaviour before members of the general public. It took no great intellectual ability to appreciate the potential advantages of the situation – which was just as well, as I had no great intellectual abilities available to me at this precise moment, thanks in part to the generous quantity of gin and tonics I had imbibed prior to the evening's ever-expanding entertainment.

Even the less well acclimatized military observers would not have been forgiven for failing to perceive that he was not cutting me down to size purely because I deserved it – which of course I did. It was undoubtedly more to do with the fact that he felt it made his current standing (inflated though it already was courtesy of discreetly inserted shoe raises) look even greater in the eyes of his now increasingly embarrassed yet far from disinterested audience.

When he had finally run out of words like 'Childish', 'arrogant', 'insolent' and 'unprofessional' he finished off with: 'I shall be keeping an eye on you, Sparrow, remember that. I shall be watching you all the time you are here.'

There is only one potent, defusing response to this threat that I know of – once you have ruled out the 'I'm terribly sorry, sir, I didn't mean it and I'm deeply ashamed,' approach. Wing Commander Colclough stood but half a pace in front of me, and I could not resist it.

I leaned forward and grasped his right hand in both of my own, shaking it warmly.

'Thank you, sir, so much,' I enthused, 'for taking such an interest. It can be quite lonely out there, and it will be so good to know there is somebody like you keeping a helpful eye on my career. Might I ask if you could do the same for a few of my colleagues? I know they would be proud to look to you too, sir, for some professional guidance and advice.'

I turned and walked briskly away, a beatific smile upon my face, leaving him to wonder just how it had gone so horribly wrong.

6

Headley and St Mawgan

From the dreary, subterranean depths of St Athan it was onwards – and definitely upwards – to RAF Headley Court, an idyllic haven of rest a short journey outside Leatherhead, in Surrey.

The first stage of my vocational general practice training was now complete, if you could call Andrew's approach vocational, and his methods akin to training.

'You had better sign this,' he said tersely towards the end of my tenure, handing me a long list of non-existent tutorials we were supposed to have undertaken.

'But . . . ' I said, running my eye down the page, 'we didn't actually have these tutorials together, Andrew, did we?'

'You want to pass?' he replied, his already less than substantial upper lip thinning itself a little further. 'Then you sign the document.'

I wanted to pass.

At that time the qualification requirement for prospective GPs was eighteen months as a trainee in a group practice, under the benignly watchful (if you were lucky) eye of a senior colleague, followed by three six-month attachments in any hospital speciality of your choice, each of these being a bold step of uncertainty into the yawning abyss of the unknown. The generally intended aim was to absorb as much of an alien branch of medicine as was possible given the stringency of the time restraints, and to try and avoid involvement in any litigation case that would re-quire your mostly 'absent without leave' bosses to accept the merest hint of responsibility for their lack of ethically defensible conduct.

RAF Headley Court was my first and decidedly foremost choice of all the opportunities available. It was a Rheumatology (inflammatory and mostly debilitating arthritic diseases) and Rehabilitation post, and I had all but begged to be accepted there.

Headley was the one mountain-top breath of fresh air in the otherwise ubiquitously spread administrative pollution I was to encounter throughout my time as an RAF doctor, and came with the added advantage of the best bar I have ever seen, or would ever wish to. Steeped in history, with an intricately carved ceiling bearing the hallmarks of two centuries' artistic endeavour together with a vertiginously patterned carpet that neatly camouflaged all recently eruptive bilious attacks, it welcomed you into its ever-encompassing embrace from the moment you first crossed its portals — and found the barman unconscious in the tap room.

Many years previously Headley had begun life as a small house in the country with large grounds, grandiose ideas and a succession of progressive owners who had each added a wing or two, or even an extra storey, in the hope of marking their passing. And the gardens . . . they were to die for.

It had begun life as a joint RAF and army station in the aftermath of the Second World War, specifically designed to cater for the needs of those often horrifically wounded servicemen who had nowhere else to go, no other hope of recovery. As the years had passed, and obviously war casualties became thankfully fewer and further between, it had expanded its remit in order to survive.

In 1986 there were only four doctors still working there, all RAF personnel: the Station Commander, a Group Captain in charge of both the whole enterprise and the separate Head Injury Unit; a Wing Commander Consultant Rheumatologist,

'Dashing' – as we called him . . . or was it what he called himself?
– Steven Tombs, whose enthusiasm for the post was matched
only by his love for the leaded-windowed town house he
occupied in nearby Leatherhead; and two junior doctors, of
whom I was one.

But it was the backroom staff who made the place what it
was, a whole supportive team of physiotherapists, occupational
therapists and in pride of place, to my way of thinking, the army
PTIs (Physical Training Instructors), some of the finest professionals it has been my privilege to work with.

There were many severely disabled patients at Headley, from
all walks of life, all types of background, including a handful of
civilians. Burns victims; those who had lost one or more limbs
in the cause of duty, or occupational pursuits; and those struggling desperately to recover from routine orthopaedic surgery
who needed the time, the input and the impressive expertise so
readily available in order to return to the demanding lives they
had previously led.

To try and put it into perspective, an accountant, say, or even a
GP such as myself, can return to his desk job with a pronounced
limp or sporting the odd crutch or two, but soldiers and airmen
returning to active duty were an entirely different proposition.
They needed to be restored to full fitness, or more, in as short a
time as possible. Ninety per cent just would not do.

Headley was in some respects like any other military base,
and in others so very different. Those patients who were officers
– and civilians accorded 'officer' status, dependent upon their
professions – lived, ate and slept (metaphorically speaking) in
the officers' mess together with the doctors and the small number
of commissioned administrative staff who manned the camp. The
non-commissioned ranks lived at the other end of the central
courtyard in mud huts with no electricity or running water,
packed in like sardines behind booby-trapped barbed wire fences
and begging for food and water from passing villagers.

The major difference about the whole camp, however, centred around the congenial informality of the place, a genuine air of working towards a common goal with a refreshing lack of the usual burdensome political red tape. We all wanted the same things: the best for our patients, to maximize their recovery to the utmost of our collective abilities, to mend their broken bodies and minds, to nurture . . . well, you get the idea.

Of all the patients I encountered at Headley there are three who remain indelibly printed on my mind.

Foremost amongst these was Ann, my great friend, whom I first encountered when she was in the throes of recovering from a terrible car accident in which she had broken more bones than I remain capable of naming, even now. Ann was a great proponent of the officially banned – and gleefully politically incorrect – 'Cripples' Race' round the officers' mess.

The starting point – of course – was the bar, from which you had to clamber up a variable number of sets of stairs before racing down the labyrinthine corridors to descend again to the ground floor via another flight. This all required a complex handicapping system based on the number of broken bones you were carrying, the amount of metalwork required to put you back together again and the weight of whatever walking aids you needed to successfully negotiate the carefully planned circuit.

Able-bodied participants had to do an extra lap, and drink more before they started.

It was sad, funny, rewarding . . . it was so many things to us all. The whole range of human emotions could be found there – despair, hope, often bitterness and defeatism, but most of all I remember the laughter, the courage in the face of adversity and some of the outrageously stupid jokes that we played on each other.

What really sticks in my craw, however, is that I never won a race – not a single ruddy one of them.

Peter was a dark-haired, ruggedly handsome army officer, a fanatical climber who had fallen down a crevasse in some far-off northern land – possibly Manchester – and lain undiscovered for a few days, almost dying of exposure. Somehow, miraculously, he had survived, but the intricate repairs to his right leg resulted in it being two inches shorter than his left, which effectively should have put an end to his mountaineering exploits.

But Peter – a combination of arrogance, humility, boyish charm and sheer, absolute bloody-minded determination – had other ideas.

Against virtually everyone's better judgement, and goodness alone knows how, he had managed to persuade an army ortho-paedic surgeon to break his good other leg and remove an equiv-alent two inches, to balance them up.

'One day,' he would say with complete conviction, 'I'll be back there, up in the mountains where I belong. One day . . .'

I would watch him some nights, gritting his teeth and limp-ing painfully back to his room from the bar, defying any of us to offer him the merest suggestion of help, the slightest hint of sympathy, and I would wonder . . .

And then there was Philip, an officer in a Scottish regiment who, as he used to say with a wry smile, had 'more metal work in my back than the Forth Road and Golden Gate bridges put together.' A succession of steel rods held his spine precariously in place, and some days just watching his agonizingly slow progress from one rehabilitation session to another was almost too distressing an experience for the observer, let alone Philip himself.

Philip, like many of the patients, was back on his third or fourth visit at Headley. As each one passed it became increas-ingly, ominously apparent that he would never be able to make it back to active service. The dreaded day finally came.

'There's nothing else we can do for you, I'm afraid,' said Colonel Southgate, the visiting surgeon, studying the latest set of X-rays. 'I'm sorry, Philip, really I am, but I think the time has come for you to leave.'

'Leave?' said Philip, struggling desperately to comprehend. 'You mean leave Headley? Another month, sir, please, couldn't you give me that? Some more time, maybe, I'm beginning to feel a little bit stronger every day, I can do more . . . Surely . . . '

He ground to a halt, catching the look on the surgeon's face.

'Yes, leave Headley . . . and, well . . . ' said the Colonel, as gently as he was able, ' . . . it means leaving the army too, Philip, I'm afraid. It's finally time to go. Much as I hate to say it, there is nothing left that we have to offer you. Nothing that will work.'

We sat up late together that night, Peter, Philip and I, long after everyone else had retired to bed. Philip, who had been drinking even more heavily than the other two of us, was all but asleep on the bar room sofa, and Peter and I were just about to finally escort him to his room when he sat up suddenly and announced, 'I need a piano.'

'A piano?' we exclaimed together.

'Yes, a piano,' he repeated, somewhat puzzled. 'You do know what one looks like?'

We nodded in unison.

'Good. I thought you probably would, being men of exshpe . . . expre . . . experience,' he continued doggedly. 'I need a piano, and I need you to take me to one now.'

We found him a piano. It seemed the least we could do.

What followed next is something I shall never forget.

Philip – who had hitherto shown not the least sign of any previous musical aptitude – sat, and played, and sang the 'Flower of Scotland' as if his whole life depended upon it. It was one of the most haunting, the most lyrically beautiful, the most poignant things I have ever heard.

I left Headley three days later.

Ann remains thankfully a friend to this day, but of Peter and Philip?

I never saw or heard from either of them again.

At the end of my six-month stay at Headley I had a three-week break prior to taking up my final posting at RAF Wroughton, one of the then few remaining military hospitals.

Oh goody, I thought innocently. An unexpected holiday.

Oh goody, thought somebody more senior than me in the postings department. A spare pair of hands . . .

I was sent, much against my will, to what then seemed to be the end of the earth but was in fact RAF St Mawgan, deep in the wilds of Cornwall and not so very far from where I now live. The single-handed doctor who was there had been taken suddenly ill, and they were desperately in need of someone mature, responsible and professionally competent to take his place.

And when they couldn't find anyone like that, they sent for me, instead.

I arrived early one evening – amazingly, the exact same evening I was supposed to – and made my way to the officers' mess to establish where I was sleeping. The mess was rather nice – nice carpet, nice bar, nice rooms – and I looked forward to spending two weeks comfortably ensconced there.

Except it wasn't there I was to be ensconced . . .

'Ah yes, Flight Lieutenant Sparrow, we have a room specially reserved for you,' beamed the mess manager encouragingly. 'Room 6B. I'll just get you the keys.'

He turned, rummaged in a filing cabinet for a few moments and emerged triumphantly holding a set of keys in his hand.

'Ah yes,' he said again . . .

(He started every sentence with an 'Ah yes,' I was soon to find out, and often wondered if he did the same at home.

'I'm afraid the cat's dead,' his wife might say.

'Ah yes,' he would no doubt reply. 'I've been expecting it.'
Or . . . 'Are you still constipated, dear?'
'Ah yes, but that new laxative's working wonders . . . ')
' . . . nice room we have for you, sir.'
'Down the corridor, near the bar, staggering distance only?' I
enquired eagerly.

'Ah yes,' he agreed temporarily, 'but in fact . . . well, no. It's
actually across the courtyard – heading south-west – around the
corner, a brisk walk of no more than a hundred yards straight
ahead and it's Block B, room number six. Ah yes, a nice sheltered
little spot.'

'Is it en suite?' I asked, maybe just a little optimistically.

He handed me the keys and smiled rather emptily. 'Ah yes,'
he said absently, adding quietly as I crossed the lobby to the
front door, 'in fact no. Not actually.'

The spill-over accommodation from the St Mawgan's officers'
mess consisted of a group of less than entirely luxurious Nissen
huts. These – for those of you strangely unacquainted with such
woefully abject neolithic edifices – are semi-cylindrical corru-
gated iron structures designed by the great Colonel P. N. Nissen
(1871–1930) himself. And they were very nice Nissen huts, as
far as they went . . . but I wish they had gone a little further.
Somewhere south of the Equator would have been good. I had
not until then realized that they were in fact based upon an
original design built initially for the Battle of Hastings, and
what stood before me was no doubt one of the prototypes –
which was subsequently dispensed with . . .

But it was dry – the warm summer breeze permeating gently
through what remained of the roof ensured that; spacious – an
impression created by the absence of any furniture; and had an
unparalleled view of the surrounding countryside through the
generous array of gaping holes in the walls.

And yet I didn't mind. All I was in need of was some food,
preceded by a drink, preceded by a change of clothes, a hot

shower and an all-over massage by something blonde, Swedish and with little inclination to talk.

I undressed, wrapped a towel around my waist, and leaving the all-enveloping luxury of my room wandered the dozen yards down the corridor to the bathroom. So far all was fine, as was the shower itself and the amble back to my room, but at this point it suddenly became very unfine indeed.

I had locked myself out.

Of course, I could have asked for assistance from any of the other occupants of Nissen Hut Block B, but sadly for my predicament – there weren't any. Or I could have rung through to the officers' mess from the B Block telephone – except that there was only one in the building, put in specially for my visit, and it was waiting patiently for me behind the very same bedroom door as the rest of my belongings. I suppose I could have just slept in the corridor in my towel, and worried about it all in the morning – but I didn't.

I walked to the mess, towel clutched firmly round my waist, crossed the empty lobby and made my way into the bar, where I hoped I might find some sign of life, and a little much-needed assistance. Which I did, in a way . . .

Two hundred guests, representatives of the county's 'Great and Good' and enjoying pre-dinner drinks before a charity evening ball, turned and looked curiously at me. Two hundred jaws, and one towel, dropped to the floor.

The mess manager drifted Jeeves-like to my side, calmly bent down, picked up my towel and handed it back to me.

'Ah yes. I suppose this is what you might call exposing yourself to the glare of publicity, sir,' he said calmly. 'Welcome to RAF St Mawgan.'

I arrived at the medical centre the following morning to sly grins all round. Naked doctors may be ten a penny in a student bar – and always male, for some unaccountable reason – but in the officers' mess at RAF St Mawgan it was something of a new phenomenon.

'Morning, sir,' said the young airman behind reception. 'I would have guessed you must be our replacement doctor, but you appear to have all of your clothes on.'

After the first couple of hours the jokes began to die down a bit, and I relaxed into my morning's work. At 11.30 a.m., on the dot, the alarm sirens sounded, and we were launched into a station exercise.

It is hard to explain the complexities, importance, and sheer mind-numbing banality of a station exercise to a civilian audience. It was completely out of the question to try and explain it to a doctor. As far as I could ascertain, it was just a really good excuse to dress up in lots of asexual green clothing, carry a gas mask whilst pretending you actually understood how to put it on in an emergency, stick a silly green hood on your head and stay away from your family for anything from a few hours to a couple of days at a time. The whole process was supposed to simulate a nuclear attack – a pretty common occurrence in Cornwall, of course – and sharpen your response time and defensive awareness.

I could never quite get to grips with how the ability to say at the earliest possible opportunity, 'Oh look, a nuclear bomb has just exploded south of Truro,' was going to help our long-term survival all that much. Equally, unlike so many of my colleagues, I derived very little vicarious pleasure from wandering around in androgynous green overalls and learning how to have a pee without exposing any part of my anatomy to the hostility of the surrounding chemically polluted environment. And in any case, I'm sure if I had wanted to there would be a private members' club in Soho where you can do this type of thing without ever needing to pretend there are bombs in the offing.

But it was pointless to resist, so in time-honoured fashion I learned to adapt and make the most of the situation. Like many RAF doctors I had quickly learned to avail myself of the medical

centre valium and sleep through as much of the experience as
was possible in our designated 'Nuclear Holocaust Beds' – in
other words, the wards, unless there were real patients cluttering
up the place. I endured my isolation with good grace, read all
the old *Readers Digest* copies with the greatest of pleasure, and
settled in for the duration.

And then lunchtime approached, and I was beginning to get
hungry. I had no doubt that the officers' mess would have a snack
or two concealed somewhere in their premises, and that after
my salutary experience of the night before they would be only
too happy to point me in its direction. It seemed entirely reasonable to me that while the rest of the station should be enjoying
the obligatory reconstituted potato gruel – all in the cause of
the protection of their country – I should be tucking into steak,
chips and mushrooms with a glass of something smooth, red
and alcoholic.

The mess was less than two hundred yards away from the
medical centre. So what if there was a silly little military curfew,
and total embargo on movement between buildings without
written permission? I was no ordinary mortal, and had never
pretended to be one of 'them'. I was the doctor, wasn't I, and
the normal rules of conflict just did not apply to me. Did they?

'I'm off to lunch,' I announced casually to the assembled
medical centre staff. There was a collective intake of breath.

'Don't really think you should, sir,' said the sergeant know-
ingly. 'There are rules, you know.'

'So there are,' I agreed happily, 'but they are for other people,
and I feel a steak coming on. Smell that mushroom, taste that
chip . . . what are rules, Sergeant Patterson, when compared with
that?'

'Rules are what other people make and we adhere to,' he
replied solemnly. 'They are what brings order to our society,
structure to our establishment, method to our madness – '

'But sadly, not lunches to our doctors, ' I interrupted pointedly, 'and somehow lunch seems rather critical, right now. I'll see you in an hour or so.'

I left the medical centre, deaf to their very sensible protestations, and strolled lazily in the direction of the mess. Oh, this was the life. The sun was shining, the birds were singing, and more importantly, I didn't have any patients to see now the exercise was in process. I could stretch lunch to a good hour and a couple of pints, and that would take me through to the afternoon session of the World Snooker Championships. Not even an RAF St Mawgan station exercise can last longer than a major snooker championship.

Half-way there I was stopped by what I presumed to be a routine guard patrol, although had I thought . . . but there was no affable 'Excuse me, sir, may I see your ID?' or 'Just off to lunch, sir? I do hope it's something succulent.'

They just stopped in front of me and said tersely, 'ID, please.'

'Nice day for a war,' I said amicably, trying to break the ice a little. 'And hey, green really suits you,' to the nearest and biggest of the three.

They stood, completely expressionless, and waved their guns at me. I tend to assume that RAF guns are like those second-hand plastic replicas you get at car boot sales, but I have to say that these were rather good copies. Might almost have been real, in fact.

I gave them my ID card. It seemed the polite thing to do. It was actually my third card – one I had legitimately lost, and the second had kindly given its life in the cause of scientific experimentation late one night in the bar when the bet was it couldn't be melted in less than ten matches (and it can't) – and I had received it only two or three weeks earlier.

I had never really looked at it, save for a passing glance to make sure the photograph sufficiently resembled me when viewed through dark glasses on a gloomy winter afternoon, and on each previous occasion I had been required to produce it, it had been passed with an unconcerned wave of the hand. Just like a credit card, really – when did the checkout girl in Tesco's last look properly at your signature? Exactly.

But these guys studied it intently, and then their eyes narrowed collectively.

'Number?' they demanded in unison.

'One of me, three of you,' I said brightly, and then caught their expressions. '5204461U, Flight Lieutenant Michael Anthony Sparrow, Caucasian, height 180 cm, eyes sort of a muddy greeny-brown, two years' service to date, and getting really rather hungry and looking forward to lunch.'

I held my hand out to retrieve my card, and suddenly three firearms were being pointed directly at my chest. Worse than that, at least one of them looked like it might actually work.

'Lie down,' hissed the first of them.

'Certainly,' I agreed readily, 'I fully intend to – but after lunch, if you don't mind. I do so hate to lie down on an empty stomach.'

'Now,' hissed the second.

The third didn't waste all that time in hissing. He just pointed his gun at my head, and twitched it slightly.

'Now look,' I said slowly and gently. 'I'm just the stand-in doctor here, I'm not in the least bit interested in your big boys' games, and I'm hungry, I'm going to lunch, and you lot may collectively go forth and multiply.'

I've always liked to think that tact and diplomacy rank high amongst my finer characteristics.

Of course, what I did not know at the time was that in the middle of a routine station exercise a genuine bomb alert had taken place. It was during the height of the IRA bombing campaign, and a suspect package had been discovered in Station Headquarters.

What I also did not know was that the person who had planted the suspected bomb was thought to still be at large on the base, possibly in possession of a false ID.

But what I really did not know was that when my new ID

card had been printed, a simple mistake had been made. Instead of the date of issue being stamped as 2/6/84, somehow it had been embossed 2/6/94, a mere ten years in the future. To the security men I was an unknown individual, with a false ID, in the vicinity of a recently planted bomb, and most heinous of all, I couldn't give a stuff about security arrangements.

They frisked me.

Not the casual way they run a hand vaguely over you whilst chatting to a colleague that you get at the airport, but real frisking, and that's when it all began to get suddenly serious.

In my top left-hand shirt pocket, below several layers of the green fetishy stuff, I had what I knew was my doctor's bleep. Sadly, what I knew was my bleep they thought was a remote control detonator for the suspected bomb in the Station Administration Centre. I thought it was a joke; they thought it was a life-threatening device, and we treated its discovery on a slightly different level.

'It's my bleep,' I said with complete honesty, reaching up to get it out and show them. 'My doctor's bleep. We all carry them.'

Three guns twitched menacingly. Three voices rasped, 'Don't touch it.'

'It's just a bleep,' I reassured them in world-weary fashion. 'It goes "bleep bleep, bleep bleep," when somebody wants me.'

'Lie down,' spat out the meanest and twitchiest of them. 'On your stomach, arms and legs stretched out as far as you can.'

In the distance, on the steps of the officers' mess, I could see a couple of officers who had witnessed my inadvertently indecent exposure the night before laughing together and pointing in my direction, obviously thoroughly enjoying this great joke at my expense. I resolved not to lie down, but to go for lunch.

'Lie down now,' said another of them harshly, in a manner that seemed to imply that maybe, perhaps, just possibly, it would be a good idea if I did.

I decided that lunch could wait. The grass looked dry, and

comfortable, and it seemed only polite to make my new-found friends happy in their work. And besides – those guns . . . They were beginning to look more and more real, and as if they might suddenly go off. I lay down cautiously.

For the next five minutes, a sort of semi-farce took place. Every now and then I would sit up and say something like, 'Now look, I've had quite enough of this, and I'm off for an aperitif,' and the guns would twitch, and I would lie down again. I could see this going on interminably, and lunch disappearing off the menu.

Nothing much seemed to be happening – I was still doing all the lying down, and they were doing all the gun pointing, and having all the fun – and eventually I decided that I had had enough. I can take a joke as well as the next man – sometimes – but I was beginning to feel that this one had gone on for far too long.

I sat up, and ignored the pointing – but no longer twitching – guns aimed steadfastly at my chest.

'For the last time,' I said slowly and evenly, 'I'm a doctor. I'm here on a two-week attachment before my next posting, I arrived last night and exposed myself to everyone of any importance in the county, and now I'm tired and I'm hungry and I don't want to play your stupid little games any more. So now I'm off. If you wish to shoot me in the back, please just fire away. I'll not hold it against you.'

I am not at all sure that I want to know what might have happened next, had not the nurse from the medical centre – a civilian, and hence comparatively immune from the rigours of station exercises and all the fun they involved – wandered by at precisely that moment.

'Hello, Dr Sparrow,' she called cheerily. 'Dropped something in the grass, have we?'

'Yes, Eileen,' I answered, without the merest hint of sarcasm. 'And these three kind gentlemen are helping me to pick it up. It's called my sense of dignity.'

The guns were beginning to lower themselves.

'You know this man?' asked one of my captors, curious despite himself.

She grinned. 'Everyone on the station apart from apparently you three knows this man,' she answered drily. 'This is Dr Sparrow. He arrived last night as a stand-in for Dr Cummings. He used to work at Chivenor – I know the nurse there. He's, er . . .' she looked at me, and winked unobtrusively, '. . . he's made quite a name here for himself, already.'

I swear my erstwhile captors were looking disappointed, although at this stage I was still not exactly sure what was going on. The atmosphere had changed completely, and they explained why they had stopped me, and taken it all so seriously.

'And you really thought I was a terrorist?' I asked faintly.

It seemed that they really had.

'And what would you have done if I'd just got up and wandered off, without the timely intervention of the nurse?'

The most senior of them regarded me soberly.

'Then I would have shot you,' he said.

A sudden chill pervaded the air, and I shivered, and then shrugged it off. He wouldn't really have shot me. Would he?

7

Wroughton, and a Little Problem with . . . Fletch

And so, finally, to RAF Wroughton, a military hospital based a few miles outside Swindon, Wilts, which would perhaps herald the closing chapter of my as yet not so very illustrious service career.

But who would have been able to predict the twists of fate that awaited me, around each and every unexpected corner?

Wroughton was then one of the rapidly dwindling contingent of bi-service (Army and Air Force) hospitals still in existence, but the sands of time have since run sadly and inevitably dry. Where people once strode the corridors in pride, vomited in the flower beds with impunity or contracted life-threatening diseases whilst visiting distant relatives on a whim and the promise of an unsubstantiated legacy, Wroughton is now no more, reduced to a barren wasteland of its former, under-appreciated glory.

As I write these words the air is redolent only with the pervading aroma of decay. Whilst the property developers rub their hands with undisguised glee the builders move slowly, ominously forward, ever eager to lay waste to a heritage that can never be replaced or rediscovered, to a past we may not revisit again, and to a laundry service that was frankly little short of despicable.

Located high on a hill overlooking the surrounding countryside, Wroughton was to be my last – and, I hope, for once controversy-free – port of call on a whirlwind tour of Her Majesty's Forces' establishments. A year hence – God and the punitive correction facilities permitting – I would be leaving on a journey of endless discovery to chart the relatively unknown territories of the outside world.

Exotic, far distant lands remained unexplored. New horizons beckoned. The M25 rose luminously into view.

But for now it was a new start, a new station, and a fresh beginning . . .

Here, at last, hopefully no one would know – let alone recognize – me. Here, at last, no one would recall my past woefully poor record of indiscipline, my almost inexcusable but undying affiliation to the claret and blue of West Ham, or even my inability to insert a catheter the right way round and into the most deserving patient.

Here at last there was surely nothing else that could go irreparably wrong. 'Please' I begged daily, 'please, not this time.'

But, as so often before, it was not an auspicious start.

Moving from one RAF station to another was a difficult enough process at the best of times.

After a year or two in any one location you would have begun to form friendships with neighbours, colleagues, local publicans, only to be suddenly uprooted, mostly against your will, to a place you had never seen and quite often never even heard of. And to make life all the more difficult, we had to suffer the iniquities of the 'marching out' process, a visitation from hell that made Dante's Inferno look like a ten-minute play session in the ball pool at the local theme park.

On the face of it, the policy seemed eminently sensible. As you left a property it was carefully inspected for any signs of damage, defects or lack of cleanliness – and all very reasonable too, you might think.

We would all of us wish to move into tidy, well-scrubbed premises, and would hope to vacate our previous lodgings upon the same basis. The RAF, however, appeared strangely disinclined to contribute to this arrangement in either financial or practical terms, which consequently meant that the last few days of any stay in service accommodation were spent reeking of bleach whilst searching the furthest recesses of the loft for rat droppings, the next-door neighbours' children and any junior member of staff who had incurred your displeasure. And if that was not enough to keep you out of mischief there was always the task of replanting your garden with all the things that your predecessors had grown but which had died during your tenure.

Like the grass, for example.

Into this feverish maelstrom of activity would stride the housing officer, the Devil Incarnate's personal envoy but with fewer redeeming features. He was invested with awesome power, and his job – no, his mission in life – was firstly to ensure that you left your house as others would want to find it, and secondly that you lost touch with what little remained of your sanity.

Can you imagine how difficult this whole process could be if you had small, sticky-fingered children running round under your feet, three different species of incontinent pets and an uncontrollable mother-in-law staying at the time?

In earlier times the position had generally been held by junior officers, usually women, but all that was to change. So many stories abounded of white-gloved harridans running their fingers along the top of doors and picture rails and howling in delight on discovering the merest speck of dust, that they cannot have all been apocryphal. Senior officers, too, had become thoroughly disenchanted by their juniors instructing them to, for example, 'Clean out that toilet again – and I suggest you use a little more bleach, this time.'

The post passed into civilian hands and all went further downhill from there, if that were possible. When we left St Athan, for example, I was fined £25 because the housing officer found a cobweb in the garage – three days after he was due to undertake his original inspection.

'But spiders need homes too,' I argued compassionately, but somehow he didn't see it quite the same way.

The nightmare over, it was time to head east, and hopefully to salvation.

As we drove up to the officers' quarters at Wroughton for the second time that morning, the sun was making a feeble effort to shine through heavy clouds after a weekend of truly abysmal weather.

Our second housing officer in twenty-four hours met us on the doorstep of our intended home for the next year, looking irritably at his watch.

'You were meant to be here twelve and a half minutes ago,' he complained. 'I've been waiting.'

'And getting very cold too, by the look of it,' I said sympathetically. 'Or are you always that blue round the lips?' I pursed my lips thoughtfully. 'Do you get chest pain when you climb the stairs? Have you had your blood pressure checked recently, or your cholesterol? And what about making a will . . . Are you well insured?'

I could see him visibly blanching. 'Shall we get on with it?' I persisted, 'whilst your health still holds out?'

I do so love my job, just occasionally.

He opened the door and I followed him in. A worrying smell of damp permeated the air.

'I see you've had it specially aired, then,' I said, maybe a touch sarcastically, as I made my way through to the back sitting room. A scene of devastation met our eyes.

A tree had obviously blown over some considerable time in the past and smashed against the living-room window. Six months of winter weather had wreaked its inevitable toll, and where once there had probably been a rather attractive carpet, there was now a rain-soaked, fungi-sprouting sodden morass.

'We can't live in this,' I said disgustedly. 'Look at it — it's totally uninhabitable.'

'But you wouldn't have to use this back room,' he said, completely taken aback. 'There's only the two of you . . . we can get it repaired.'

'You're absolutely right,' I agreed fervently. 'You can get it repaired, and we don't have to use it – because we won't be in it. We are not moving in here.'

'But you have to,' he persisted. 'It's the only Flight Lieutenant's house available on the officers' patch.'

'Do you know something?' I responded, looking him squarely in the eye. 'I don't care if it is the only house available in the world. I – we – are not moving in here. Nobody would. By the way . . . ' I added as a thought crossed my mind, ' . . . when was this place last inspected? Not recently, that's for sure. But isn't it your job to make sure that all accommodation is fit for each and every member of the RAF to move into?'

He opened his mouth to speak, and closed it again without having come up with an answer.

'And in any case,' I continued, smiling sweetly, 'we arrived here about an hour ago, and took a quick look round the patch, trying to identify which house we'd be staying in. Now, that one over there, for example . . . ' pointing across the road to a rather splendid edifice I had noted on our earlier reconnaissance trip, 'that's empty, isn't it? And oh look, there's my furniture van turning the corner down the road, right on cue. Where would you like me to tell it to park?'

'Not there,' he said, shaking his head virtuously. 'That's a Wing Commander's house, that is. You can't have that one.'

'Why not?' I persisted. 'Is there a Wing Commander currently living in it?'

'Well, no,' he admitted lamely, before putting on his best Jobsworth hat and rallying briefly to quote chapter and verse, 'but you can't have it anyway. No officer is allowed to occupy a house designated for a rank two or more higher than his own.' (I was then a Flight Lieutenant, and between myself and the

144

exalted position of a Wing Commander was the small matter of a Squadron Leader.)

I had been in the RAF too long now to be fazed by such behaviour.

'I see,' I said, stroking my top lip thoughtfully. 'Now, let me explain carefully. My name is Flight Lieutenant Sparrow, and I'm sorry . . . ' extracting a notebook and pen from my top pocket, 'you are . . .? For the record, you understand, not to mention my official complaint. Now, given the state of your waistline and the receding nature of your hair, I would imagine you have been employed by the Air Force long enough to appreciate a few of the basic facts.'

A glazed look was beginning to pass across his face.

'You will, I am sure, know,' I continued undeterred, 'that doctors in the Air Force are promoted from Flight Lieutenant to Squadron Leader not – thankfully for some – according to merit but strictly on account of the number of years service. After five years, the whole process is automatic. And my five years is up . . . ' I took a cursory look at my watch. 'Oh look, today! What a fortunate coincidence. Here is my ID card, should you be in need of any proof,' thrusting it unceremoniously in his face, 'which will unequivocally demonstrate the accuracy of all I am saying to you. So I want to move into that house, now, unless you wish to answer to the Station Commander within the next twenty-four hours as to why you have so grossly neglected your duties in respect of this derelict hell-hole of a residence, why you have failed to treat me with the respect my new-found rank deserves, and how you intend to pay for the rent of my furniture van for the next four months until this house is rendered duly habitable.'

It was no contest, to be honest. We moved in within the hour.

'Are you really due to be promoted today?' asked my ex, during one of the few conversations we still had with each other.

'Not actually today,' I grinned. The spectre of Belize (see *Country Doctor*) was still hanging over my head. 'In fact not actually at all, unless I behave myself for the next six months. But he wasn't to know that, was he?'

Wroughton had its faults, but to my way of thinking it was a good, old-fashioned hospital in a way rarely seen these days.

We treated patients, quite simply, according to their clinical needs – as opposed to some external political diktat. The Armed Forces' medical ethos was constructed around the system of triage – and OK, it might have come from the French, but one can't discriminate against a good idea on those xenophobic grounds alone, much though we would all ideally wish to.

Triage, reduced to its simplest terms, went as follows. Treat the patients who are in imminent danger of dying straight away; treat those who might die within the subsequent forty-eight hours next; and patch up the walking wounded as best you can between coffee breaks and bonding sessions.

Hospitals have changed so much since I last worked in them, now some fifteen years ago. Matrons have gone, and with their demise have come declining standards due to the loss of so much of the discipline which I firmly believe every ward needs to run efficiently. Each ward used to be like an extended family unit, where everyone knew everyone else and the job each was required to do. My only recent experience is as a patient, courtesy of a back in need of emergency surgery, and I swear half the staff would have been unable even to recognize the other half, let alone refer to them by name.

There are now so many more specialities, as well, some of which I can scarcely pronounce. Gone, by and large, are the general physicians and surgeons who could turn their hands to pretty much anything within their sphere. Now there are physicians specializing in hearts, or lungs, or livers . . . surgeons who deal with only vascular problems, or bowels, thyroids, even bladders and prostates. The list is endless – I await the appointment of the Britain's first Professor of Ingrowing Toenail Surgery, and you probably think I'm joking.

146

Is this just the inevitable march of progress? Am I being some sort of reactionary Luddite, a role I thoroughly enjoy when you shove a computer in front of me and ask me to use it for administrative purposes I am completely unable to fathom? Are any of us in the health service any better off for the multitude of changes we have all had to deal with in the past fifteen years?

The answer, I think, is that we can do more, but we often actually achieve less. The longer I have been in medicine, the less time I spend doing what I was originally trained for, and what I hope I still remain best at – sitting in front of patients and trying my utmost to deal with their problems. I have transformed, chameleon-like, into a part-time businessman – an uneasy combination of manager, accountant, health and safety officer and the bloke who empties the bins when my staff and the dustmen are on strike.

Like I suspect the majority of currently practising doctors I am conservative with a small 'c', but it's the big 'C' fraternity I blame for our present predicament. The longer New Labour remain in power, however, the more I – like an increasing number of my colleagues – begin to despair of their ever getting things right, as their ideas regarding improving the health service seem to be formulated according to a Bob the Builder mentality.

'With this I can fix it,' says Gordon Brown, waving a big cheque tantalizingly in our direction.

Oh, if only it was that simple. Doctors are mostly balanced, apolitical creatures – we dislike and despair of all politicians on an equal and rational basis – and just want our health service back, to run as we think it should be, not they.

It never used to be like this.

In the first big revolution to modernize the health service in recent times, back in 1991/92, the Conservatives instigated the drive to inspire competition between 'rival' hospitals. Under this Machiavellian system hospitals received payments according to the number of referrals and admissions dispatched in their direction over a set period of time. It was, inevitably therefore, greatly in their financial interests to maximize these. The more operations they undertook, for example, and the quicker the patient throughput, the more they got paid.

Given the choice, as a pressurized hospital manager, which would you prefer – ten quick and easy operations, like hernia repairs, for example, or one long, complicated and expensive one? Would you rather send a patient home a day or so earlier than clinically recommended to balance the books, or keep them in until they have fully recovered and risk running into the red? This is scarcely the most exhaustively critical analysis of the health service you will ever read, but even from my thumbnail sketch I hope you will be able to see that what is good for the hospital is not necessarily what is in the best interests of the patient.

It's what I call 'Think Tank' medicine. Whereas doctors research, evaluate, audit and endlessly reassess all that we do, I suspect that most health policy is formulated by politicians with limited medical experience or understanding after a few hours of indiscriminate brainstorming over a canapé or two. Judging by the standards of the last decade or so there have been precious few brains involved and a serious lack of constructive storming. At best, the result is the germ of an untested ideological change in the entire system probably written on the back of a cigarette packet, then to be launched upon us deeply cynical GPs to put into practice the best way we can.

But hey, what do I know? Why should anyone countenance my views, just because I've been involved in medicine for the past twenty-five years? What possible reason could I have for thinking that I, or any of my far more experienced and better educated colleagues, might have insights into our profession that would elude a newly appointed cabinet minister with his previous three years' experience as a second reserve under-secretary in the Foreign Office?

I met, during my time in the RAF, one of those very same cabinet ministers, a man who had just been elevated to an important position in the Ministry of Defence yet knew as much about Her Majesty's Services as I do macramé. I encountered him again four years later in Okehampton, a local town in Devon, when he came down to explain the rationale behind the new GP contract. He had been in the Department of Health for less than a month, and spent two uncomfortable hours hiding behind an oily smug smile and a batch of political minders trying unsuccessfully to disguise his disturbing lack of knowledge and understanding of all we were being required to do.

How can we have confidence in such people, irrespective of their political persuasion? How can we respect those who so ineptly assess our needs, and those of our patients, expecting us to undertake so many time-consuming, mind-numbingly boring paperwork exercises that will never, *never,* save one child from abuse or one lonely, desperate patient from an early grave?

And how can I hope to descend from the ever-increasing height of my soap box without risking some sort of fatal injury . . ?

Another casualty of our 'new, improved' (makes it sound like some sort of washing powder, doesn't it?) systems was the long-standing tradition of what we still refer to as 'one-stop' medicine. This, a rather imprecise but nonetheless generally more effective approach to time management, had worked something like this.

Imagine, like myself, you are a handsome, intelligent . . . well OK, somewhat rumpled and defeated rural GP encompassing his mid-life crisis with some relish when you are called out in the middle of the night to see a woman in her late thirties with severe abdominal pain. The decision as to whether she will require hospitalization or not is often easily made, but determining the precise diagnosis of her symptoms, in a badly lit cottage somewhere in the middle of the outer reaches of nowhere, can be tantamount to impossible.

The underlying cause of her complaint might ultimately prove to be surgical, gynaecological, urological or any number of other unanticipated medical causes. You make a wild stab in the dark — sorry, clinically evaluate the patient on the basis of your comprehensive knowledge of their past medical history, their current signs and symptoms and the volume of their screams — and admit her under what you feel to be the appropriate speciality.

Every once in a while you might actually get it right.

But let us suppose you have not.

The patient enters the hospital under the care of the surgeons, and her abdominal pain settles during the course of the night. The surgeon, after a full evaluation of her condition from the tranquil security of the doctors' mess, decides that the morbidity of her problem probably falls outside the limited remit of his domain.

'She needs an ultrasound,' he declares solemnly, after consulting the support cleaning staff, 'followed by a gynaecological opinion.'

In times past, the surgeon — as I have done many times myself — would make his way down to the ultrasound department and begin pleading his case with the on-call radiologist to fit her in before she went home. He would also ring the on-call gynaecologist, or chat to him over lunch, and ask him to pop down to the surgical ward to give an opinion. Having duly visited, if the gynaecologist then thought that it was perhaps a urological problem and the patient needed a further X-ray, the whole process would be repeated again.

The patient may well spend an extra day or so as an in-patient than she might otherwise have done, but she would at least be more likely to leave the hospital on her ultimate discharge with a provisional diagnosis and all the relevant speciality assessments and investigations having been undertaken. At worst she would have a properly thought out treatment plan and an organized follow-up regime.

But nowadays?

Let us assume again that the patient largely recovers overnight. In our new world, as we know it, she will be discharged the following lunchtime with a handwritten, often barely legible carbon copy note to her GP suggesting she should be referred back for a gynaecological opinion and whatever further investigation is deemed appropriate. A full typewritten discharge letter will follow when the recruitment and staffing problems have been sorted out in the typing pool, which is a bit like saying, 'The cheque is in the post.'

What then follows is another external referral, another clink of the hospital cash register and another undisclosed bonus in the hospital manager's pocket. But if the poor suffering patient meanwhile needs an ultrasound, she will have to await it as an outpatient. In the exorbitantly elongated interim the patient and her hapless GP – in this case myself – are left to pick up the pieces, staring glumly at each other across my desk with no diagnosis available, no proper plan for treatment, and no idea what to do if she has a recurrence of her pain whilst we are waiting for a final assessment.

And all of this for the sake of a phone call to a colleague, or a trip of maybe a hundred yards down a hospital corridor. It is frustrating, it's inefficient, it leads to all sorts of unnecessary delays and often further suffering for the patient, but most of all . . . it is plain wrong.

Wroughton was old-fashioned in another respect too – its construction. It was arranged essentially round one great long corridor which ran the entire length of the building, with wards coming off at right angles on either side. Simple, efficient . . . and mostly falling to bits.

The first six months, as a junior physician, were quiet and peaceful, passing with little in the way of incident. The only event of note I can recall was when a young soldier of about nineteen was admitted for investigation of a very low blood count.

After all the routine blood tests, X-rays, etc. the consultant, a Lieutenant Colonel, decided that the next step should be a rigid sigmoidoscopy – inspecting the area of bowel just above the rectum (from the inside, of course). To undertake this required, logically enough, the use of a rigid sigmoidoscope, a foot and a half of cold steel which brought tears to my eyes the moment it arrived up from the stores and he unwrapped it lovingly in the nurses' office.

As he advanced down the ward like a pikeman in the Cromwellian army, brandishing it proudly in front of him, there was a collective gasp of dismay from all the conscious patients on the ward, at least three of whom lapsed into immediate comas from the shock of the sight. Each patient held their breath until we passed by the end of their beds, sighing then in utter relief as they realized their rectal canals were safe from any form of barbaric invasion – for today, at least.

At the far end of the ward, in the very last bed, sat Private Fredericks, his eyes fixated upon the ever-approaching instrument of torture like a startled rabbit caught in the glare of oncoming headlights. Captured for all time in my mind is the look on his face as we passed the bed before his, the last vestige of hope, and the final hint of colour drained from his face as the dreadful truth hit home.

Yes . . . this was for him.

So the first six months passed without any great incident. But the next six . . .

Why is it the telephone never rings in the middle of the night during a bad dream?

I have a recurring nightmare from which it could awaken me with the greatest of pleasure, but somehow it never seems to oblige. I am seventeen, and my mother wakes me early one morning.

'It's you're A levels,' she says, handing me a cup of coffee. 'They've brought them forward a bit.'

'How much is a bit?' I enquire sleepily.

There is a pause while she considers the logistics, and then, 'Not a terribly big bit,' she answers at length. 'Just a matter of three months or so.'

'Which means, roughly?' I yawn, slightly bored with the conversation by now.

'Which means roughly – get dressed this instant. Your father's already in the car, waiting to drive you to the first one right now . . .'

A huge gaping pit opens in front of me. It's that same feeling you get when England are about to start a penalty shoot-out with Germany, when the cricket commentator says, 'Only thirty runs to get, seven wickets in hand, and the Ashes are ours for the first time in a quarter of a century,' or you open your eyes from the deepest of sleeps wondering why a policeman is standing in your room, and then you suddenly realize that you are actually asleep in his . . .

But I never get woken at this point. It is always when England are about to score that critical penalty, or make that winning run with all seven wickets still in hand, or when the policeman turns out to be a policewoman after all, and she's turned up at my eighteenth birthday for no other reason than to take her clothes off. Yes, that is when the phone inevitably rings, and you launch yourself into the merciless abyss of reality.

It is three o'clock in the morning, howling a gale and pouring with the sort of rain that we haven't experienced for a generation. As consciousness is slowly regained you remember with a sinking heart that you are an obstetrician in the RAF, you're on call, and you have to crawl out of bed. Not only that, but you forgot to fill your car up with petrol last night, so you have to creep over the fence and abscond with your neighbour's youngest daughter's bicycle and hope fervently she's grown out of those training wheels by now . . .

The midwife's voice spoke urgently in my ear. 'Mike, wake up and get here as quick as you can. I've just delivered a baby I don't like the look of. It's colour's all wrong . . . hurry, please!'

I leapt from my bed, threw on some clothes, headed for Chloe's (my neighbour's daughter) bike – yes, still with the training wheels on – and pedalled through the wind and the rain as fast and furiously as I could.

I arrived at the hospital entrance in a matter of minutes, gasping for breath and soaking wet from head to toe. After glancing carefully around – you just never know who might be watching at 3.30 in the morning – I hid Chloe's bike (with now just the one remaining training wheel) behind the privet hedge to the left of the front door.

I was safe. No one had seen me. I breathed a sigh of relief and walked into reception.

'Hello, sir,' the young man behind the desk greeted me smartly. 'Another little trip on Chloe's's bike for you, was it then?'

I nodded shamefacedly.

'Still with the training wheels on?'

I nodded again.

'Glad to see you didn't fall off, sir,' he continued jovially, 'you riding without your body protectors and all. Those little abrasions can be so painful, can't they?'

I nodded once more, and then stood back. 'Hang on,' I said thoughtfully, 'am I not the officer here, and you the senior aircraftsman?'

'Quite right, sir,' he agreed.

'Then doesn't that mean I get to use the sarcasm at your expense, and not the other way round?'

He considered this proposition carefully for a moment or two. 'Well, you are a doctor, sir, and normal rules don't generally apply in your case but, seeing as it's you, sir, go right ahead.

Feel free. Ready when you are, sir . . . ' He waited for a second or two. 'Anything particularly biting coming through yet?'

'Oh . . . bugger off, Johnson,' I said good-naturedly.

'As you will, sir. Now, on your way to maternity, are you?'

'No, Johnson, just came into the hospital at this ungodly hour in the morning for a little breath of fresh air.'

'Right, sir,' he continued, undeterred, 'then would you be so kind as to show Lance Corporal Jones the way, sir, if you wouldn't mind?'

He motioned to the young, well-built soldier a few yards behind me whom I had until this point failed to notice, and who had been following the exchange with a bemused look on his face. 'Welsh Guards, sir,' whispered Johnson by way of explanation. 'They respect their officers there, they do.'

'Do they indeed,' I rejoined. 'I wonder what that's like. Come on then, Corporal Jones, off we go.'

We jogged the fifty yards or so to the maternity department and burst in through the doors to find an empty waiting area.

'Hang on, Corporal, I'll find someone to help you,' I said. 'I presume you're looking for a wife, with or without a baby, something like that.'

'Er, yes, sir,' he said hesitantly. 'Something like that.'

I made my way to the delivery suite and pushed through the double doors, where a scene of urgent activity met my eyes. The midwives, both of whom I knew well – night after night of watching *Prisoner Cell Block H* in the nurses' coffee room together forges a bond that time can never cast asunder – were in a state of extreme anxiety, bent over a newly arrived scrap of humanity with worried frowns on their faces.

'Thank God you're here,' murmured Susan, the nearer of them. 'There's something wrong, Mike, I don't know what it is. Heart seems OK, he's breathing all right, but it's his colour, it's all wrong. We've given him oxygen, checked his airway, done everything, but he just won't go pink.'

I glanced across at the baby's mother, a young blonde girl with concern beginning to etch across the fatigue, relief and pride already present on her face, and then back to the baby, eyes screwed up tight against the first light he had seen.

'What do you think?' hissed Jenny, the second midwife. 'What's wrong with him? What shall we do?'

I drew a deep breath, composed my features, and said authoritatively, 'We'll ask the father what he thinks, shall we?'

'Mike, have you taken leave of your senses — what little you have left of them, that is?' asked Jenny, aghast. 'You're the doctor. Aren't you even going to look at him?'

'I can see him from here,' I said, 'and he looks just fine to me.'

'Look, Mike,' she snapped, 'normally I can go along with your arrant stupidities because mostly you seem to know what you're doing. But this time . . .'

I raised my hand to stem the flow. 'Have faith, my child,' I grinned, 'and meet Corporal Jones.'

I opened the door and the good Corporal, who was pacing the corridor just outside, turned and strode into the room as I beckoned, a look of keen anticipation on his face.

The midwives' jaws dropped.

'Oh,' they said softly together, as the very large, very happy and very black Corporal Jones picked up his newborn son, who was neither blond, nor pink, but a wholly reassuring shade of coffee brown, and cradled him gently in his arms.

Whilst on duty in an RAF hospital one was supposed to wear a certain form of regulation clothing. It was commonly referred to as a uniform.

Some people — and I have met them — would all but iron their shirt, polish their shoes and press their trousers even if summoned to an emergency Caesarean at three o'clock in the morning, all the better to present the finer face of the Air Force to the general public in their hour of need.

156

Me? T-shirt and jeans, generally, or whatever was nearest the bed, and hope that when you got to the hospital at least most of it was actually yours. As far as I am aware, the majority of patients in the aforementioned hour of need do not give a stuff what their doctor is wearing, as long as it is devoid of other patients' bodily fluids, doesn't give off too much static electricity and covers the greater part of the unattractively bulging bits. What they really want is a doctor who knows what he is doing, rather than one who is the epitome of sartorial elegance but stands quivering in the corner with a vacant expression on his face.

With Corporal Jones' son now safely delivered, happily looking precisely the colour God had designed him to be, I crept quietly away to the front door and the gloomy prospect of a return trip on Chloe's bike. Which is where my troubles began . . .

My bleep went off, and I groaned.

'No rest for the wicked, sir,' said Johnson, grinning broadly as he passed me the phone through the hatch.

'Apparently not,' I agreed mournfully. 'Still, look on the bright side.'

'Which is, sir?' he asked.

'I'll be needing someone to take Chloe's bike back for me,' I said, straight-faced, watching a look of horror spread over his features.

A flurry of incoming admissions to the maternity ward kept me busy all night, and at nine o'clock in the morning I was still there, delivering away frantically in the company of the midwives, who were as always wonderful in every respect.

Babies are like that, even more so than London buses. None ever seem to want to emerge blinking into the world in the daylight hours, or during a party political broadcast, but come the opening credits of *Match of the Day* or the witching hour of two in the morning and suddenly they're dropping like flies all over the place.

So when my consultant – whom I shall avoid naming out of respect for . . . out of respect for . . . oh, to hell with it, his name was Fletcher – arrived on the ward, I was marginally less than ideally attired.

He, of course, was his normal impeccably dressed self, hair neatly combed – both of them – shoes so highly polished you could have turned the lights down and white coat that must have lived in a Chinese laundry for weeks upon end.

I, on the other hand, was wearing a Meat Loaf sweatshirt which was no longer completely new, frayed jeans with holes in both knees that owed more to the time since their manufacture than a desire to follow the current trends, and a pair of trainers that had passed their 'wear by' date many years previously.

He regarded me in that singular manner I have been known to encounter from other senior doctors in the past. It eschews the elements of pity and plumps straight for exasperation, distaste and single-minded ferocity in an interesting display of conflicting emotions. If I were ever to have my throat ripped out by a Dobermann Pinscher then this is precisely how I would expect it to look as its jaws opened in mid-pounce, preparing for lunch.

'And what,' thundered Group Captain Fletcher, 'do we have here?'

I was very busy, and I was very tired, and I was just not in the mood to be shouted at, which did not bide at all well for the most diplomatic response available – and which probably explains why I didn't give it.

'It's a maternity ward, sir. Thought you might have recognized it, you being a senior gynaecologist and obstetrician and all. It's where all the local women come in the full throes of labour, secure in the knowledge that expert professional help is but a stone's throw away at all hours, no matter what the time of day or night.'

Strange how you sometimes seem not to know the most prudent moment to stop. I was on a roll. 'You might try coming here every now and then, sir, in the wee small hours. It's a friendly place — good company, lots of interesting noises, little wiggly pink things that we in the trade refer to as babies …'

I stopped. Not solely due to the look on Fletch's face, or because the ward sister was sneaking behind the filing cabinet as protection against the incipient volcanic eruption, or even because David, my counterpart junior obstetrician (who worked for one of the other consultants), was stamping surreptitiously on my foot and mouthing, 'Shut up, Mike, for God's sake.'

I stopped because I just could not be bothered to go on. I had been on continuous duty for forty-eight hours, with less than ninety minutes' sleep. I had been midwife, obstetrician, paediatrician, physician … I had even swabbed the floors on a couple of occasions, and not once disturbed my consultant from his slumbers.

I will gladly accept criticism when it is due. Well, all right, I will sometimes grudgingly acknowledge adverse comment when I am unquestionably in the wrong. This, I have to say, did not seem to me to be one of those occasions.

'How dare you,' exploded Group Captain Fletcher, 'come on to my ward dressed in such a fashion? How dare you?'

I opened my mouth to reply, and then closed it again as the ward sister, now hiding behind Fletch's back, went down on bended knee, hands clasped beseechingly together and mouthed, 'Don't hit him, Mike. Please God, don't hit him.'

'You have had more warnings about your behaviour than any other senior house officer in my memory …' said Fletch menacingly.

'Oh goody,' I said brightly, unable to contain my excitement at such glad tidings. 'Thank you, sir, that cheers me up no end.'

Kathy, the ward sister, raised her eyes to the heavens, and kept them there. 'Hopeless,' she muttered, 'absolutely hopeless.'

'… and warnings,' continued Fletch, surprisingly oblivious to my interjections, 'obviously don't mean anything to you at all, so some sort of action is now required. I will not have such complete, unmitigated insubordination from junior officers. I want you off my ward now, and I don't want you to come back at any price, Sparrow. Do you understand me? You are a liability that is just no longer worth bothering with.'

The ward became eerily quiet, the sister's office cocooned in silence. I stood, and I thought, and then finally I spoke.

'Why don't you,' I began slowly and evenly , 'just . . . '

Kathy, still cowering behind Fletch's back, shook her head vigorously. 'Please don't,' she whispered again. 'Please . . . Please don't.'

' . . . just . . . ' I repeated slowly.

David hacked viciously at my shins, catching me painfully on the ankle. 'Don't,' he grunted, turning it ostentatiously into a cough as Fletch's evil eye slid briefly over him and then returned lizard-like, unblinkingly, to me.

' . . . just . . . do the work yourself, then?' I said mildly.

I turned, left the office and walked casually down the corridor without a care in the world. Well, sort of.

As I reached the corner and disappeared from their view, I leant my back against the wall and slid slowly to the floor, exhausted.

I could have grovelled. I could have apologized, explained, pleaded and even begged – probably any one of them would have done, and all of them together would have been perfect. I could even have asked for written testimonials from patients, colleagues, my mother, or the elderly woman I had met at the supermarket the day before who had dropped all her tomatoes on the floor and was so very grateful when I picked them up for her . . .

I could have done any of those things, and probably still have had a job.

But I didn't.

We all have our own personal character flaws, and I like to think

160

how grown up it is of me to readily acknowledge mine. Of course, I have to simultaneously concede how ridiculously childish it is of me to continually follow a course of action that so frequently lands me in scaldingly hot water, following which I usually fail completely to take the appropriate remedial action.

I think this somewhat blinkered approach to life can be summed up succinctly in just the two words – one of which is 'pathetic', and the other 'stupid'. I have this sad tendency to think it more important to make a point than to consider the consequences of doing so, which is invariably to my long-term disadvantage.

It generally goes something like this.

When I was sixteen I was selected to play football for the senior under-eighteen county side. This, I have to reluctantly admit, was quite an honour, as I was the youngest player at the time to have been chosen and the grammar school I went to had previously displayed a disdainful approach to the eleven-a-side game, playing only rugby up until that term. I was, in truth, rather proud of this achievement, but would not have admitted it for a moment. To anyone.

As I was actually quite a good soccer player, and knew it, and probably easily the best centre forward they had – and sadly knew that too – I felt this excused me completely from adhering to the same rules of county representation as did everyone else. And yes, with the benefit of nearly thirty years' hindsight I too think it childish, and arrogant, and stupid, and wonder what on earth I thought I was playing at.

So when they said 'Please turn up at 9.30 . . . ' (for an 11.30 kick-off) ' . . . to discuss tactics,' well, I didn't. Who needs to talk tactics, for goodness sake, when it is all so simple? You just kick the round leather thing into your oppositions' net more often than they kick it into yours and the odds are, you'll win. Easy, isn't it? All of which explains why, when the rest of the team were earnestly discussing how to defend at corners, counter attack at speed and pull your opponents' shirt without being spotted by the referee, I was still fast asleep in my bed, living only five minutes' walk from the sports ground.

I duly arrived at 11.15 – bags of time to spare, I thought happily – strolled casually into the changing rooms and looked confidently for my number nine shirt – which I eventually found after a few minutes' frantic searching. Unfortunately, for some reason I could not then immediately comprehend, it was adorning somebody else's back at the time. How could this possibly be?

'Sparrow, you're late, and you're the substitute,' said the coach tersely as I stood looking forlornly at the number twelve shirt, which was the only one not currently having a body wrapped inside it.

'But . . . ' I began, feeling rightly humiliated. 'But what?' a small voice said in my ear. 'But you are better than Thompson, but twelve is your unlucky number, but it wasn't your fault that you were late as an earthquake disturbed an unexploded bomb at the end of your street first thing this morning . . ?'

'But nothing,' said the coach shortly, and I do believe he was actually not interested in me, which was infinitely worse than being cross. 'Maybe this will teach you a long overdue lesson and stop you behaving quite so much like a prima donna in future.' And then he rubbed my nose in it as hard as was humanly possible. 'But knowing you – I doubt it.'

This was sadly so accurate that I had no witty response to hand, no bitingly sarcastic rejoinder. There was no alternative but to flush an unattractive shade of dark red and sulk for a bit, after which I followed meekly behind as the rest of the team – those that were actually playing, as opposed to me, who wasn't – ran out on to the pitch. I walked moodily to the touchline, where I stood even more moodily throughout the first half, and an awful lot of the second, taking my punishment like a boy.

The opposition's coach obviously had the same idea about tactics as had I, because by midway through the second half they had kicked the round leather thing into our net on four separate occasions, and we had deposited it in theirs . . . well, we hadn't in all truth deposited it in theirs at all.

I have no idea as to whether our coach would have considered my humiliation complete at this point or not, but the situation was resolved for the pair of us when the occupant of 'my' number nine shirt wrenched his knee in a tackle and was unable to take any further part in the game. My great moment had arrived. I trotted out on to the pitch with not the least bit of enthusiasm for the thankless task ahead, and took up a position midway inside our opponents' half before noticing that my bootlace was undone.

And this is where fate decided to lend a hand, offering me the irresistible chance to cut off my nose in order to spite the entire rest of my face, if I should choose to take it. As I started to rise, bootlace now duly tied, I heard the coach bellow, 'Wake *up*, number twelve, look for the ball, will you?' and at precisely the same time I saw the round leather thing arrowing its way towards me at waist height, following a defensive clearance by our centre-half, like a Cruise missile in search of an Al-Qaeda stronghold.

What happened next, unless you are a Michael Owen or Thierry Henry, comes around only once in a career. With my back to the opponents' goal, and a defender snapping at my heels, in a blur of movement I trapped the ball on my thigh, flicked it over my own and the defender's head with my right foot, ran round behind him and volleyed it into the top corner of the net with my left foot from fully twenty-five yards.

I don't know who was most surprised – me, the coach, or the opposition goalkeeper, who just stood and looked at the ball as if he couldn't quite understand how it had got there. Even I was impressed.

With my first touch of the ball I had scored the goal of a lifetime – mine, at least – undoubtedly guaranteed myself selection for the rest of the season, and probably earned a chance to progress up the ranks to better and better representative sides. All I had to do was to capitalize on my stroke of good fortune, in a mature and dignified way, and make the most of it.

I wandered, however, casually to the touchline, where the coach was standing with a mixture of frustration and grudging admiration on his face, and took off my shirt, throwing it across to him with a careless 'Thanks for the game.' Stunned, he watched speechless as I walked off the pitch, into the changing room and out of a future in football.

The whole thing had taken less than a couple of minutes.

My actions on that day of course demonstrate the strength of character of a young man of unquestionable personal integrity and principle. Or do I mean the infantile stupidity and arrogance of an immature boy who should so definitely have known better, but sadly did not?

My point in recounting all this is my firm belief that you take your character, flaws and all, and the lessons you learn from the school yard all the way to your medical school, and from there out into the big wide world as whatever sort of doctor you might ultimately become. Study your GP, or consultant, and there you may still see the inadequacies of youth, all badly papered over with a couple of degrees and a long white coat. Those flaws will ooze out all over the place, making a right mess on the carpet, if you just wait long enough.

Your job is just to pretend that you haven't noticed.

There is a constant game played in the world of medicine, with ever-shifting goalposts but some firmly established rules:

Rule 1: Be obsequious to your superiors at all times, especially those who will shortly be writing an appraisal upon you and thus determining your professional future.

Rule 2: Get as many letters after your name as you can. Any old letters will do, as few people even in the medical profession have the least idea what most of them stand for.

Rule 3: Publish. Publish anything at all, as long as it has some sort of medical slant to it. 'A randomized double-blind trial into the constituents and rate of production of ear wax' would suffice. And don't you worry – no one will ever get around to reading it, but it will look awfully good on your CV.

Rule 4: Develop a complete lack of concern about your professional competence. It is as irrelevant to your ability to progress in your chosen career as is your degree of vocational dedication and what your next-door neighbour's cat eats for dinner. Provided, of course, you follow Rules 1 to 3 assiduously.

There was a time when – if you did not wish to play by the above rules, or progress appreciably up the medical hierarchy of life – there was a simple way out, a universal escape route. Anyone could do it.

The answer? Become a GP and disappear into a quasi-respectable obscurity. Training? References? No need to bother with all that, for goodness sake, that's for those stuck-up 'proper doctors', them as what works in 'ospitals.

We GPs could bumble away happily in suburban anonymity, dealing with the odd dangerously heavy cold, an acute, life-threatening case of acne or a strange smell emanating from your grandparents. As long as we didn't polish off too many patients in the first month or two – which was by no means a guaranteed state of affairs – our careers, and more importantly our future income-earning potential, were made for life.

But not any more. Those halcyon days are long since past, and sadly people now expect us to have some vague idea as to what we are doing for more than fifty per cent of the time.

So when the choice ultimately arises between one's principles and one's career – as sooner or later it almost inevitably will – and when no accreditation in your present training post means no future qualification as a GP, and therefore no job, or even the prospect of one, to be had, what on earth is one supposed to do?

The following week at Wroughton was rather pleasant, in many respects.

I didn't have to get up early, and I didn't have to come home late – because, of course, I didn't in fact have to go to work at all.

My nights were blissfully undisturbed, except by the dog's digestive difficulties. I slept the sleep of the just, and the pure in heart. For seven whole days the prospect of no job seemed infinitely less important than the prospect of no sleep. And anyway, I consoled myself, something would turn up. Something usually did.

Meanwhile, in strict contrast to my week of leisure, news was beginning to filter through from the hospital. Fletch, bless his little cotton socks, was apparently starting to wilt under the strain of having to work for a living, and bets were being cast as to how long he would last. At RAF Wroughton each obstetric consultant had but the one junior member of staff, and Fletch's junior member of staff was . . . me.

So if I wasn't doing my job, it meant that he had to. If I wasn't spending night after sleepless night patrolling the wards, then once again it meant . . . he had to. And if I wasn't spending day after meaningless day dealing with the routine paperwork, taking the routine bloods, clerking all the routine admissions, dealing with the emergency deliveries and examining the newborn babies, then . . . well, then *he* had to, of course, and in addition to all of his own work, too.

Poor chap. He was a consultant, after all. He shouldn't have been bothered with all those menial little tasks that we underlings did uncomplainingly for him day after day, week after week, as a matter of course . . . like emptying the catheter bags when the nurses were all busy playing three card brag in the boiler room. What is the point of being an overling if you have to knuckle down to a proper bit of work, just like everybody else?

'He's looking very tired,' reported David, dropping in on his way home one evening. 'He was admitting a patient, one of his "due for a Caesar the moment they start asking for a lawyer" cases, and he kept forgetting to ask her all the right questions. And I'm sure he overheard Kathy muttering, "Flight Lieutenant Sparrow would have done it in half the time" to me, and he didn't even have the energy to shout at her.'

'Goodness, he's that stressed, is he?' I said, as sorrowfully as I could manage under the circumstances. 'I think I'm beginning to sympathize with him.'

'No, you're not Mike,' said David solemnly. 'I know you, remember, and you don't really sympathize with him at all.'

Things were looking good. And when Kathy rang me the next day to say, 'He fell asleep in the office this morning, and then thanked me when I woke him up and brought him a cup of coffee,' I just knew most of the omens were on my side.

All I had to do was to sit, and to wait, and to bide my time.

Ten days into my Fletch-imposed exile the hospital registrar called round to see me at home.

The registrar, usually a senior doctor, occupies an odd sort of position – part government whip, part trouble-shooter and junior doctor's ally against the powers that be, and part clinical policeman. He is in many respects the oil in the lumbering wheel of hospital machinery, easing the often less than smooth running of the wards.

We had met mainly, to date, in his capacity as a sort of head prefect, a duty which required him to gently rebuke those junior doctors who had inadvertently stepped out of line. Most junior doctors survived their fledgling careers without ever being summoned to the equivalent of the head prefect's caning, but he and I had finally come to a mutually acceptable compromise.

He introduced the revolutionary concept of the 'FBS', as it later became colloquially known, which followed strictly pre-established guidelines. I would enter his office and salute smartly – a difficult concept for me to grasp, but one that I soon became used to – and he would motion for me to sit down. I would then remove my cap, always provided I had remembered to put it on in the first place, and meekly take my seat as directed.

'Well, Flight Lieutenant Sparrow,' he would begin sternly, 'welcome to your Fortnightly Bollocking Session. Any major sins you feel compelled to confess since our last meeting together?'

'No, sir,' I would respond solemnly.

'Good,' he would continue. 'Then for the sins you have recently committed, the sins you are no doubt currently committing, and the sins you are absolutely guaranteed to commit before we next meet, consider yourself well and truly pardoned.' (He confessed to me one day that it was a good deal easier to just turn a blind eye to my transgressions than to have to actually think about what punishment he would eventually be required to apply.)

'Thank you, sir,' I would reply gravely.

'Well, that's all over then,' he would say, visibly relaxing and pushing across his cigarettes and lighter. 'And thank goodness for that. Now then, Mike – better hang on for another ten minutes or so, make it look a bit more official.'

And raising his voice to his secretary he would call, 'Hi, Janet, formalities over. Any chance of a cup of coffee?'

'I must be going up in the world,' I said as I opened the door to him, 'if I've graduated to home visits. Business, pleasure, or gin and tonic?'

'All three,' he sighed, entering the hall and crossing through to the living room, where England were for once contriving not to lose to the Australians – but only because it was raining. 'God, it's a pleasure to get out of the office.' He nodded towards the

168

television. 'I suppose you've been sitting watching a lot of that for the past ten days.'

'I suppose I have,' I agreed happily, 'and I suppose I've been rather enjoying it, too.'

We chatted inconsequentially for a few minutes and then the Registrar – Wing Commander Brian Hicks, to give him his due title – drained his glass and looked across at me, suddenly serious and obviously not knowing quite where he should start.

'Well, come on then, Brian, which is it to be?' I asked quietly. 'Death by a thousand cuts or salvation in the form of Fletch's conversion to Christianity? The glorious and unexpected resurrection of my not yet entirely glittering career, or the unemployment office in the morning?'

'Mind if I smoke?' he asked, breathing out heavily, and I shook my head, offering him a light. He inhaled deeply and blew out a steady stream of smoke, watching it intently as he said, 'It's actually in your hands, Mike. But I know you're not going to like it.'

I shrugged, far more nonchalantly than I felt. 'Well, it's not going to be the first time I've got myself into a position like this,' I said, 'and pretty unlikely to be the last. Go on then, Brian, spit it out – I'm a man, I can take it.'

He turned away, surprisingly hesitant for a man of his general bluntness and common sense, and stood looking through the living-room window at my dog, who was entertaining both herself and Chloe with what remained of my RAF beret.

'He's prepared to accept your apology tomorrow morning,' said Brian at last, 'and if you are equally prepared to comply then he will consider the matter closed. He gets his junior member of staff back, and starts to sleep nights again, and you get your reinstatement, your accreditation, and your career. He feels that that is more than a fair exchange.'

'I see,' I said, feeling my teeth begin to grit. 'So all he wants is for me to apologize to him for rushing into work in the middle of the night – in an emergency, need I remind everybody – in a hastily put on pair of jeans and a sweatshirt and being too busy to go home to change into my uniform before he wanders in bright and bloody breezy after the full night's sleep I've allowed him to have by being bloody efficient at what I was doing? It doesn't seem to have occurred to him to apologize to me for having acted so precipitately in throwing me off the ward I was bloody well running for him under the most difficult of circumstances, having been up all night without a moment's rest. And not content with that he then threatens to ruin my career, but he wants *me* to apologize to *him?* I don't think so.'

'That's about the size of it,' agreed Brian, with another of his sighs. 'Of course, you wouldn't have been in any way rude, or insolent, or "couldn't care less about his seniority"-ish in front of any of the other ward staff. Would you?' he added.

I remained quiet, trying unsuccessfully to appraise the situation in a cool, balanced manner.

'Of course you wouldn't,' continued Brian, his voice dripping with irony. 'That's not the sort of thing you ever do at all, is it? Come on, Mike, think about it. Swallow your wretched principles for once in your life and apologize to the man, for goodness sake. Keep your fingers crossed behind your back if you must, but do it, please. What is more important to you? Your career, your future livelihood, the ability to feed both of your dogs without raiding the next-door neighbour's dustbin again – or what you still insist on referring to as some pathetically outdated sense of principle? Possibly the only person in the northern hemisphere who has even the merest inkling that you might be right in what you are doing . . . is you. Welcome to solitary confinement.'

'Oh, come on, Brian, that's not fair.' I turned to the window and stood looking across the fields at the hospital. 'It's too late for me to do anything else, and besides, I can't in all honesty say that I want to. Level with me, Brian – we both know that Fletch has been getting away with this sort of behaviour for more years than probably even you can remember. Sooner or later someone has to make a stand or he'll go on and on, pushing and shoving all the junior staff around as if they don't matter a damn. We're all just the most ordinary of people, remember, doing the best that we can – making the intermittent mistake, I grant you, as I know that I have for one on various occasions – but there comes a time when somebody has to turn round and say that enough is enough.'

'Then let that somebody be somebody else,' Brian pleaded. 'You've got a wife and two dogs to support, and one day hopefully even children. At least if you do things Fletch's way you have half a chance of managing it. And besides, it's not just you that's involved in all this, despite what you might think, isolated on that "Little Englander's" island of yours. You might think of it as "your" power struggle, and "your" high-minded stubbornness, but other people are suffering in the fallout too, in many ways more than you are. Their careers matter to them as much as yours does, even if you've long forgotten you're not the only important person in this godforsaken hospital of ours.'

He handed me back his glass, and made to leave.

'Thanks for the drink, Mike. And please, think about what I've been trying to say to you. I'll see you in the morning, one way or another.'

I lay awake most of the night, finally dozing off in the early hours only to come to with a start as dawn was breaking. I sat by the window then, watching the minute hand as seven o'clock became eight, and eight o'clock nine. Fifteen minutes later I made my way down to Fletch's office, and a date with destiny.

Several other visitors had arrived after Brian, mostly junior colleagues but surprisingly even one of the other consultant obstetricians, all offering the same well-meaning advice. Career before principle, every time. You can always get another set of principles tomorrow.

I also had quite a few phone calls. The most interesting – and unexpected – came from Germany, and Josie, a West Indian theatre sister with a wicked sense of humour whom I knew well, having worked long hours with her in the hospital operating theatre before her posting abroad only two weeks previously.

'News travels fast,' she said, giggling infectiously down the phone, 'except when it's you, when it positively gallops along. Still need me to keep you out of trouble, I see, even when I'm a couple of thousand miles away. Couldn't have you sacrificing your career for the sake of your stupidly misplaced pride, now could we?'

We never met again, but Josie – should you ever read this, even though it may one day be in your dotage – if you have never received your reward in this lifetime, then surely it must come in the next.

Our conversation came back to me as I stood outside Fletch's door, steeling myself for the ordeal to come. As I raised my hand to knock, Kathy scurried down the corridor and clutched my arm.

'Now, you're going to do it,' she said firmly. 'You're going to apologize to him, grovel a bit if you have to, and maybe shine his shoes if they haven't been attended to for the last half an hour or so. Aren't you? Look me in the eyes now . . . '

I looked her in the eyes as requested, and grinned. She sighed audibly, like a mother whose wayward son has kicked his football through the next-door neighbour's greenhouse window again but who has run out of the energy to scold him.

'Oh my God, you're not going to do it,' she said faintly. 'Are you? Thank goodness I only ever had to work with you . . . '

Alone in the corridor once more, after Kathy's departure, I took a deep breath, raised my fist, knocked on Fletch's door, and entered . . .

Fletch was sitting behind his desk, ostensibly reviewing some notes, although we both knew otherwise. He declined to look up for a couple of minutes as I stood there, uncommonly quiet and still, with the only noise to be heard the rhythmical turning of the pages he wasn't reading before him.

Time passed equally slowly for us both, but eventually he took off his glasses, laid them carefully upon the desk and leant back in his chair. He regarded me impassively, stroking his chin with that long right index finger of his which had been in all sorts of interesting places, sometimes even with gloves on.

'Hope you've . . . ' I stopped, bit my tongue, and reconsidered. ' . . . had a good day, sir,' I concluded, though I still think I should have finished with my formerly intended, 'washed your hands carefully.'

He scowled at me over the rim of his glasses, reminding me of a cobra surveying its prey unblinkingly, just awaiting the moment to strike.

'Well, Flight Lieutenant Sparrow,' he said finally, gravel-voiced. 'Just what is it you have to say to me?'

There are some things that should remain for ever secret – but this is not one of them. Yet save for a West Indian sister in a German hospital later that night, who shrieked and whooped and hollered with laughter for some time after we had spoken together, the following has been kept from the general public . . . until this very moment.

I took a deep breath, and remembered all the advice I had been given.

'Yes, sir,' I began, 'I just want to thank you for giving me this opportunity . . . '

To my surprise, I saw Fletch beginning to relax. It had never occurred to me that he might be as keyed up as I was, and for the most fleeting of moments I thought there might be a remnant spark of humanity lurking beneath that malevolent exterior – but happily the feeling soon passed. I took another deep breath, and moved on.

' . . . of apologizing to myself on your behalf. I know the words would stick in your throat, sir, and I would never wish you such unutterable discomfort. And besides, what would become of you were you to choke, when there is only me here in a position to save you?'

Fletch's face was a picture, when I had the odd moment to observe it, a look of absolute thunder being kept at bay only by sheer astonishment at the words he was hearing.

'Let me do it for you,' I continued, preparing to burn every boat I had ever been even vaguely connected with. 'Flight Lieutenant Sparrow, I would just like to say how appallingly I have treated both you and all your illustrious predecessors. I abhor my behaviour in misjudging your admittedly unconventional attire on the ward ten days ago, and have been unable to sleep due to the shame I so fervently feel for having vented what is left of my spleen upon your entirely undeserving shoulders.'

I took a quick look across at my tormentor in waiting, and prayed that he would wait some more. If I didn't finish now, then I knew I never would.

'I acted in haste,' I continued for him, 'and on realizing my mistake – as I'm undoubtedly sure you did, sir, didn't you? – I should have reinstated you at once, and apologized sooner. Instead of which I threatened your career, and the future happiness and prosperity of all those children you have yet to conceive and are so much looking forward to.

'I can only ask you to accept my belated – but unquestionably most sincere – apologies, and beg you to consider the matter closed for both our sakes.'

Fletch had stopped stroking his chin by now, and the look in his eyes was not one you would wish to behold for too long in a non-intoxicated state.

'Anything else you wish to add?' he asked, ominously polite.

'Yes, sir,' I nodded, turning for a second as I thought someone was pounding on the door, until I realized it was my heart beating uncontrollably in my chest. 'I would like to say that I accept your apology without reservation, sir, and applaud you for giving it so freely. I can only . . . '

I ground to a halt.

'Shut up, Sparrow!' bellowed Fletch angrily, unable to contain himself any longer. 'Shut . . . ' he caught himself just before losing complete control. 'I think you've said quite enough. If there is nothing else . . . '

And then he saw the look on my face, and stopped, probably for the first time in his life wondering what he had let himself in for.

There is nothing like being in complete control of a difficult and demanding situation, and medicine can be a career like no other for putting you there, just when you least expect it.

The balance of power had suddenly changed, and we both knew it.

'Well, sir,' I said finally, 'it has come down to just you and me, here in your office with no one to bear witness. Take a look at me – no, not the maverick individual you so obviously despise, but the junior doctor who has hauled your scraggy arse out of so many difficult situations you have never even been aware of. We all sweat unappreciated blood for you and your like-minded colleagues, because it is what we are paid for, and how we get our references, but loyalty only goes so far. In the end, you need me and my junior colleagues more than we will ever need you, but it has taken a disaffected malcontent like me to make you realize it.'

Fletch, like an undiscovered volcano, was beginning to rumble.

'You've got it so wrong,' I continued dispassionately. 'You see, it's not my career on the line but your own. If you fail to sign me up I will pursue you through every court and industrial tribunal you have ever heard of, and some of which you won't. Every day you wake up I will be outside your window, clamouring for justice and denigrating your wife's dress sense. Every night you go to bed I will be there in your nightmares, piercing your heart with slivers of ice from the mortuary attendant's freezer. Whenever you walk down your corridors of power, I will be there behind you, out of sight and out of reach. All it takes to see the back of me for good, all it will ever take is your signature, right now, on that form on the table in front of you.'

Perhaps I should have been triumphant, but in truth I was just tired, battle-weary and in need of a drink.

'Sign it, sir, and I will be on my way. But if you are looking for a fight, you can count on me to give you one.'

'Supposing,' I said, as I rang Josie later that night, 'he had called my bluff? What would I have done then?'

There was a silence at the end of the phone for a few moments.

'Well, if suicide is not an option,' she said finally, 'I would have had to lend you my exhaustive directory of compromising photographs.'

'Meaning?' I asked, agog.

'It's a bad line, Mike. May I call you in the morning?'

The line went dead, and the morning – like tomorrow – never came. And I have no idea whether Fletch achieved his ultimate goal of professional recognition, or sank in the political quagmire of failed, over-the-hill non-entities. And I never cared.

One day, I like to think, we will all get what we deserve – but could I please postpone my just desserts until tomorrow?

8

The End Game

So, my long-awaited certificate of vocational training was looming fast upon the horizon – as was the spectre of unemployment.

My six-year RAF commission was due to expire in less than four months' time, and I had yet to land myself a job out in the real world. By coincidence, the day after my final denouement with Fletch my belated promotion arrived, together with a rather handsome cheque for six months' back pay.

'Squadron Leader Sparrow,' I said out loud as I looked down at the envelope. 'Rather a nice ring to it, that.'

Which set me to thinking . . .

Maybe a career in the Air Force wasn't that bad after all. Sure, I'd had my fair share of unfortunate experiences – in fact, come to think of it, rather a lot of other people's shares, as well – but wasn't it . . ? Could it not possibly have been . . ? Had it not really been very much my fault, if I'm honest, and not theirs at all?

Life as a civilian seemed suddenly full of uncertainties. I started to weigh up the pros and cons.

What did I currently have?

A secure job, if I behaved myself – a difficult one that, but wasn't it time to do a little growing up? – decent affordable housing, the prospect of financial help with any future school fees, a good working environment with plenty of support staff . . . My God, it was beginning to look positively attractive, and I hadn't even got as far as guaranteed time-linked promotion and, most important of all, the knowledge that I would be sent away from home on a regular enough basis to make life almost acceptable.

And on the outside? No job as yet, no house, no regular

income and no one to polish my shoes when I left them outside the door.

It was time to make some serious decisions, but mostly . . . it was time for some serious interviews.

'I beg your pardon,' said the OC (Officer in Charge of) Admin, looking up sharply from the paperwork on his desk.

'I'd like to apply for a permanent commission, sir,' I repeated.

'Is this some sort of a joke?' he asked brusquely. 'Because if you're wasting my time –'

'No, sir,' I reassured him. 'Not a joke – it's just that I've been thinking. Re-evaluating my life, if you like to put it that way. Look, sir, we both know I have hardly been the best of officers . . .'

'You can say that again,' he agreed, rather too easily for my liking.

' . . . but even I can change. It's only now that I'm facing the prospect of leaving the RAF that I've begun to appreciate what it is I'm going to miss. It's a good life here, sir, full of good people . . . '

OC Admin's face was a picture. I ploughed on doggedly, undeterred.

' . . . and I've come to realize that all those forms and procedures, all those tried and trusted practices and disciplinary measures I've reacted so badly to are there for a reason. I've always thought of them as restrictive, as suffocating until now, but I'm beginning at last to see the error of my ways.'

'You and me both,' said OC Admin sceptically.

'No, listen to me, sir,' I pleaded. 'They're actually rather liberating, in a funny sort of way, freeing us from the shackles of doubt and uncertainty. It's taken me an awful long time to reach the place where I am now, sir, but don't you see? If I can reform my ways, then surely anyone can?'

'Now that I do agree with,' he said forcefully, but he was weakening. I gave him my most sincere smile in return.

'Look, Squadron Leader Sparrow,' he said, after considering

for a few moments. 'Do you really mean this, because it will be your head on the block shortly after mine, if you don't?'

I nodded, temporarily unable to speak.

'Well, it won't be easy,' he warned. 'There are far too many people around here – in fact, there's an awful lot of people around pretty much most of the Air Force – who have long since written you off as the worst form of serial trouble maker. The general consensus of opinion is that you are someone we will all be glad to see the back of.'

'I know that, sir,' I admitted, shrugging with what I like to think was an air of endearing humility. 'And how can I say anything other than that I've richly deserved it? But give me a chance, sir, please – it's all I'm asking. Give me the opportunity to make some amends. I'll willingly jump through any number of hoops to show you, to show everyone that I mean what I say.'

'Well,' he said slowly, 'if you're sure.'

'I am, sir,' I confirmed. 'I can't quite explain why, but I just know it's what I want to do.'

'Well,' he repeated, 'sadly – or maybe luckily, for you – it's not just me you have to convince. I'd best make you an appointment to see the Station Commander, and soon, I suppose. He's away on holiday next week, and you haven't that much time.'

'If you would, sir, I'd be grateful. I won't let you down.'

'You'd better not,' he warned ominously. 'Mind you, you'd probably be wise to prepare yourself for a disappointment. He might be a fair man, the CO – after all, he supported your promotion on technical grounds, despite the fact he feels you don't deserve it for a moment – but there's another problem you'll have to deal with.'

'Which is, sir?' I asked tentatively.

'He doesn't like you,' he said.

'Ah, is that all?' I sighed in relief. 'Well, never mind, sir, then it's up to me, isn't it?'

'He's a hard taskmaster,' he continued, watching me shrewdly, 'but he's a God-fearing man of deep and committed Christian principles, and he'll give you a fair hearing.'

'Do you think he might pray for me, sir?' I asked diffidently.

'Oh, he'll be praying for something,' he agreed solemnly. 'You'll find it difficult to get his support, but if you do . . . it could take you a long way from here . . .'

'Thank you, sir,' I said, rising and shaking him firmly by the hand. 'Thank you very much indeed.'

' . . . and the further away the better,' he muttered under his breath as I left.

Three days later . . .

'I feel born again,' I said simply. 'As if I have suddenly seen the light. It's almost as if it has been out there all this time, just waiting for me to find it.'

'Are you a church-going man?' asked the Station Commander, a sudden gleam appearing in his eye.

'I haven't been, no, sir,' I admitted, shamefaced, 'and I'm sorry to have to own up to it. But do you know, sir, last week I attended a service for the first time in years, in the village. It seemed a bit strange at first . . .'

I looked up, hesitating, uncertain how to proceed, but gained confidence on receiving a quick nod of approval in return.

'But the service was warm and reassuring . . . strangely welcoming, as if it was aimed only at me, but I wasn't quite sure whether I felt ready to take communion, though when the time came . . . it just felt right. I was at peace. I know it sounds stupid to say it, sir, but it was like I had come home, after so many years away. I can understand you might be a bit sceptical, sir, and if I were in your position I'm sure I would feel the same, but I'm asking you to trust me, to put your faith, your beliefs into mine. I'm asking you to give me my life back.'

He was wavering, I could see he was wavering.

'I opened my Bible when I returned home,' I continued, my

eyes beginning to water, 'and I read something that has sustained me throughout these difficult times. "There is more joy", sir — and I'm sure you could finish the quotation for me — "in one sinner that repenteth" . . . '

The following week found me in London.

'It's been a long time, Mike. I guess, had anyone asked me, I would have suspected you might have been dead by now. But rumour has it you want to apply for a permanent commission,' said Wing Commander Hookman doubtfully. 'You . . . *you* want to apply . . . '

'Yes, I know, sir,' I agreed. 'It's a bit unexpected, isn't it?'

'Mike . . . ' He paused for a moment, obviously struggling for words. 'I have known about you ever since the day you entered medical school — anyone who ever went to Mary's has. I even met you once, not that you were in a fit state to remember. And I've had so many regular updates from Martin' — his younger brother, a student in the year below me — 'that I feel I know you almost as well as I know myself. You and the RAF are quite a long way from being ideally suited, which is probably the most polite interpretation anyone could ever put upon it. What on earth do you think you are doing?'

'Come on, sir . . . sorry, John,' as he held up his hand in self-deprecation. 'Have you never been a bit of a hell-raiser in your time? There must be the odd blot on your collective copybook.'

'Yes, but it's not totally obliterated like yours,' he said, elevating his eyes to the heavens.

'Well, thank you for that unexpected vote of confidence,' I murmured. 'Look, I'm sure we could both tell each other a few stories about our respective times at Mary's, yet consider you now — a pillar of every community, in a position of immense responsibility and still encompassed somewhere within the boundaries of being a real life human being. What wouldn't I give to have your job — juggling the careers of every doctor in the RAF, going home every night at three minutes to five to your wife, your children and all those video recordings of *Emmerdale Farm*? It could be me, John, a few years down the line. It could be me.'

'So what happened to the Mike Sparrow we all used to hear about?' he asked disbelievingly. 'That last bastion of independent bloody-mindedness we all so hated to admire?'

'I grew up, John,' I said honestly. 'I grew up and became like everyone else – doesn't it inevitably become the fate of the best and worst of us? And,' I added, stripped to the bone, 'I think I'm in need of a job.'

'I'll sign your forms,' he agreed reluctantly, 'if that's what you want me to do. But it gives me no pleasure to do so . . . '

There were other tiers, other interviews, other hurdles to negotiate. But gradually, step by step, I made my way to Hertfordshire, and the last stop in my hierarchical journey to meet the man on whose decision my future would depend.

I walked in with my head bowed.

'So, Squadron Leader Sparrow,' said Air Vice Marshal Guthwaite, a man I had met previously only on my ignominious return from Belize. 'I see you have a promotion to your credit.'

'As apparently do you, sir,' I responded in kind, 'since we last met. My letter of congratulation is no doubt somewhere lost in the post.'

He raised his eyebrows over some expensive half-moon glasses.

'I see the passage of time doesn't change the man, or the attitude,' he said, struggling unsuccessfully to restrain a smile. 'So tell me, Mike . . . I can call you Mike, can't I?'

I had this vague recollection of having been here somewhere before . . .

'Sir,' I responded, 'I think right now you can call me anything you want to.'

'OK, Mike, and let us avoid all the bullshit. What the bloody hell are you doing this for?'

It had been so hard, so difficult at times, but yet so ultimately rewarding.

At each escalating interview I'd had to adjust my approach, alter my perspective and change into a complete set of new underwear. But not one of the people I had met – not a single one of them – had questioned my intent, my integrity or my resolution to work harder. So entranced were they by my unexpected sincerity, so staggered by my inexplicable, chameleon-like change of heart, so warmed by my 'on the road to Damascus' conversion and the knowledge that I had finally seen the error of my ways, that they never once considered, never once thought . . .

'So, Mike, have you had a lot of fun doing this?' asked Air Vice Marshal Guthwaite.

'Oh yes, sir, I do believe I have,' I admitted with a grin.

Maybe the Air Force wasn't such a bad choice of career, after all . . .

'Then bugger off back to where you came from,' he said emphatically. 'The RAF doesn't need you, and it probably never has. But I'll tell you something else you should always remember . . .'

I opened my mouth to speak, but thought the better of it.

' . . . you don't need the RAF either. And you never will.'

So, it was farewell – at last – to Her Majesty's Royal Air Force.

Farewell to the mindlessly petty administrative banalities of Chivenor; to the boredom of St Athan, the career-threatening excesses of Belize. Farewell to the one true camaraderie of Headley, and the final moment of truth at Wroughton.

Farewell to a life of controversy and discontent, to hairline decisions on which so much depended, to bucking the system just for the sheer hell of it, and welcome . . . welcome at last to the peace and the quiet of Lifton.

Life as I had known it was over. It would all be so different now, so very different.

Wouldn't it?

9

Lifton – The Early Years

So this, at last, was what it had been all about, what I had been waiting all this time finally to do.

Six years at medical school, twelve punishing months as a junior doctor in the NHS, and a further six years in the RAF. How quickly, on reflection, the time seemed to have flown.

1 August 1988 . . .

I awoke early and walked through to the spare bedroom, taking a seat by the uncurtained windows. My gaze swept across the pile of builder's rubble that would one day become my front lawn, beyond that to the empty country lane at the bottom of the drive and up, further up to the front door of the large house immediately opposite my own.

Talbot Lodge, my new place of work. In a matter of hours I would at last join the single-handed practice of Dr Margaret, a local institution who had lived, worked and quite frankly terrified most of the incumbent population here for the past thirty-four years.

'How on earth did you get the job?' one of the local GPs asked me some time later. 'Half the unemployed profession around here have been trying to land it for ages – I even tried it myself, for a couple of years, but never so much as got a look in.'

'Ah,' I replied seriously, 'but did you ever threaten to let down her tyres and smash all her windows if she didn't employ you?'

It says something about at least one of us that for several minutes he took me for real.

The story of how I came to be in Lifton is told in my first book, and I will not here revisit old ground.

Lifton, for those of you who remain unacquainted, is a small village nestling in an idyllically quiet countryside valley just a couple of miles east of the Devon/Cornwall border. Undistinguished in many respects, its main claim to fame resides in its being the origins of the one and only Ambrosia factory, home of a million or more tins of custard and creamed rice.

In 1988 the practice had around 1800 patients spread over a ten-mile radius into the surrounding rural areas – a busy life for one GP, but a fairly leisurely existence for a partnership of two. Over the forthcoming years it was to grow, develop and change almost beyond recognition, but here and now it seemed to offer the perfect life, the answer to all my prayers for the future . . .

By 8.15 I was washed, dressed and had tied my own shoe-laces. By 8.30 I had breakfasted, and by 8.45 the valium was beginning to work. I was ready. I took a deep breath, reknotted my tie several times – each of them a little more untidily than the one before – and made my way proudly across the road, relishing the challenge ahead.

My first surgery. My first chance to get to know some of the patients I would hopefully be looking after for many years to come, my first real exposure to the country practice I had so long yearned to undertake. I stood out in the morning sun beaming down on the gravelled surgery car park for a moment, took a few deep breaths to steady my nerves then crossed to the door of the waiting room.

Another deep breath, and then opening it, I stepped in.

It was packed to the point of overflowing; hot, steamy and full of excited morning chatter – which stopped at the very moment they saw me.

'Morning, everyone,' I said, a noticeable tremor in my voice.

'Morning,' came the collective response, as twenty pairs of eyes scrutinized me closely.

'Ooh, it's him,' I heard someone whisper as I made my way down the short corridor to the consulting room. 'The new doctor. Doesn't he look young?'

'And ever so nervous,' somebody else replied in hushed tones. 'Do you think he'll turn out to be any good?'

They weren't the only ones wondering that, I thought wryly. I knocked on the door and let myself in, to find Dr Margaret in the process of taking an elderly lady's blood pressure.

'Hello, Michael,' she said, looking up briefly. 'What was it you wanted?'

'Um,' I said, taken aback. 'Well, as it's my first day here I'd come to do morning surgery, to be honest. I thought we had arranged that.'

'It's Thursday,' she replied pointedly. 'I've always done morning surgery on a Thursday, even when my late husband was alive. No point in changing too many traditions just yet, don't you think?'

'Er, yes, of course,' I agreed hesitantly, 'but, um . . . what shall I do, then? Would you like me to dispense some drugs for you?'

'No, Mrs Northey and I will do that at the end of surgery,' she replied patiently. 'Just like we always do. Why don't you come back at lunchtime, and we'll see if we can find some work for you to do then.'

'Right . . . yes, of course. That will be fine,' I burbled. 'Sorry for interrupting . . . sorry . . . '

I turned round, and making my way back through the gauntlet of the waiting room found myself out in the sunlit car park once more, less than a minute after going in. There was nothing else to be done other than retrace my steps and return home, somewhat deflated.

This was not quite the start I had envisaged.

At 12.30 I was back in the waiting room, which was now thankfully empty.

'She's gone off on visits,' called out Mrs Northey from the small reception area. 'She said would you like to come back after evening surgery, about seven, for a chat. She always does –'

'No, don't tell me,' I finished off for her with a sigh. 'It has to be "evening surgery on a Thursday." No doubt even when her husband was alive.'

'That's it,' agreed Mrs Northey, cheerfully unaware of the irony in my voice. 'I think you're beginning to get the hang of it now.'

It took time for us both to adjust, understandably.

There was I, newly out of training and still a little green about the gills but bursting with enthusiastic ideas and a whole variety of potential innovations, and there on the other hand was Dr Margaret . . . Significantly older, vastly more experienced and respected in the community, yet so very set in her ways. Looking back, I'm sure she must have found herself irritated at times by the medical equivalent of an untrained young puppy snapping impatiently around her heels.

Fresh from the cutting edge trauma of Wroughton I found the tranquillity of rural practice life initially difficult to contend with, but gradually we both adapted and moved on. Six months down the line we had both more or less found our niche, and for the next two and a half years Margaret – who had a daughter she rarely saw, working as a vet in the north – treated me, albeit in a rather Edwardian fashion, like the son she had never had.

'And neither wanted nor would have coped with,' someone told me drily, several years after her death.

We developed a pattern of alternating surgeries, shared visits and an acceptance of each other's diametrically opposed approach to general practice, whilst the relaxed, countryside tolerance I soon grew to love settled over us like a warm blanket on a chilly autumn night. Once or twice a month she would invite me into the inner sanctum of her drawing room after evening surgery, where we would sit over a glass of sherry discussing the patients we had seen. Occasionally she would offer me one, too . . .

This was, however, the comparative calm before the storm.

As you might expect, living in the small village where you practise as a GP has its disadvantages.

Your life becomes no longer your own, and living immediately opposite the surgery, initially such an apparently good idea, turned out to be a great mistake. Margaret had always operated – indeed thrived upon –an 'open house' policy, and patients would often bang on her door at any hour of the day or night. In her later years, following her husband's death, it was probably only that which kept her going, a feeling of complete indispensability amongst her human flock, but for me . . . when off duty, I wanted to be dispensable, thank you very much indeed.

Of course, living a stone's throw from the surgery did have its compensations. It took but a minute to get from home to work, and I even toyed with the idea of constructing an aerial runway from my bedroom window to the waiting room door, thus cutting down the time further. As I write, however, I cannot actually think of any others, but maybe they were there somewhere, if one were only to look hard enough.

Village life, as I quickly learned, is so very different from a city existence. You never see any foxes, for a start – they're all too busily occupied in the towns and housing estates, raiding the bins. Village people are different, too. They deal with things in a different way.

Margaret had a tremendous sense of discipline – which contrasted rather neatly with my tremendous lack of it – and over the years had applied it rigorously to her patients. The surgery opened at nine o'clock in the morning – not a minute before – and closed wherever possible on the dot of six in the evening. Outside these hours, although she would remain on call as detailed above, it was strictly for emergencies only. The countryman's definition of an emergency, by the way, is someone who is going to die just after you arrive on the scene, and just before the ambulance does.

One day, when Margaret was on one of her rare visits away from the practice to have the rod of iron reinserted in her back, the surgery phone rang at one minute past nine.

'John Endacott here,' announced a voice in a soft Devon burr. 'My mother's had a fall and broken her hip. Could you come round sometime this morning and take a look at her?'

Not 'Come round now,' as often demanded by a certain type of patient with a pain in their little toe for almost the past five minutes, but 'Could you come round sometime this morning?'

I thought I probably could.

'Of course,' I replied. 'Are you quite sure she's broken her hip?'

'Quite,' he answered simply. 'She said so.'

I quickly drove the half a dozen miles to the family farm, and found Mrs Endacott sitting up primly in bed, looking surprisingly pink and comfortable. Sure enough, her right hip was indisputably broken – how could I have ever doubted their word? – and I made the appropriate calls to arrange for her to go into hospital.

As I put the phone down after talking to an obviously exhausted young house officer who had no doubt been up most of the night, a thought suddenly struck me.

'You didn't actually break this in bed, did you' I asked curiously.

She fixed me with a gimlet eye. 'No, young man,' she said, slightly tetchily, 'but you wouldn't have expected me to lie out in the garden all night, now would you?'

She had, as I discovered after further questioning, tripped and fallen in the farmyard garden at five minutes past six the previous evening, and, hearing the cracking of the bones in her hip as she landed, knew immediately what she had done. But this, as I am so often reminded, is Devon, so summoning therefore a couple of her sons she instructed them to carry her up to her bed, thereby to await the opening of the surgery the following morning.

For fifteen hours she had lain there, in continuous uncomplaining discomfort, and at the start of the sixteenth hour she had allowed her family to request some medical help. Nobody, apart from myself, thought there was anything in the least unusual about this, because . . .

They do things differently, in the country.

Margaret, despite being slight of stature, had an undeniable presence about her. I described her in the first book as being physically not unlike the Queen, and certainly as her health began to fail the aura of regality surrounding her seemed to intensify.

Yet when the occasion sometimes demanded, she could be positively intimidating.

Our local district hospital, in Launceston, is rarely to be found as the meeting place of the unruliest of the neighbourhood malcontents, but even it has its moments.

Margaret, as was her habit, walked into the casualty department one afternoon in search of a broken bone or two to wrench back into position only to find herself quite unexpectedly in the midst of a major skirmish. A motley collection of the indigenous youth of the day had gathered to await one of their clan being sutured back together and were arguing over . . . well, I don't suppose anybody could remember, by then, or even really cared.

By sheer chance I had arrived a matter of seconds earlier on an alternative mission, and was already engaged upon planning my strategically diplomatic solution to the problem. This, I hoped, would avoid a potentially dangerous escalation in the already precarious situation, but in the final event it was obvious I was viewing it from an entirely different perspective.

There were, to my mind, only two imperative issues I should seek to address; namely which of the multitude of protagonists should I hit first, and with what, followed by which direction should I run away in immediately afterwards?

Margaret, to my complete surprise, instantly appreciating how the land was beginning to lie, strode forcefully into the midst of the affray. I watched, spellbound, from behind the safety of my riot shield whilst preparing to unleash my government issue tear gas canisters as she swept imperiously aside the inevitable collection of second-hand plastic bricks and decaying soft toys that lay upon the nearest table and climbed on to it.

'Young men,' she announced in a quiet but distinctly authoritative voice, peering unforgivingly over the rim of her glasses, 'this is a hospital, not a rugby scrum. There are seriously ill patients in their beds only a few yards from here, patients in need of peace, of quiet and tranquillity, in order that they may survive their mostly life-threatening conditions. If you continue in this utterly disgraceful vein of behaviour the death of at least one of them may soon be on your hands, and I, who have lived here for so long, have no doubt I can later identify each and every one of you to the local constabulary should,' she added darkly 'it prove to be necessary.'

I wanted to initiate a round of applause, but Margaret had yet to finish.

'Please now leave the building at once,' she continued haughtily, 'and take up your cudgels elsewhere.'

To my amazement the fighting and brawling ceased abruptly, and the bloodied, bruised and bellicose youths filed docilely out of the door. I stood in undeniable admiration, and can remember that feeling still. Oh, to have such powers of control. Would my day ever come?

And then 'What's a cudgel?' I heard one heavily limping combatant mutter to another on his way out. 'Because I don't want to leave mine behind.'

As Margaret's retirement approached I turned my attention, inevitably, towards my future survival.

I had the land on which to build a new surgery of my own,

the outline planning permission to proceed and the incipient duodenal ulcer that went with it. What I did not, on reflection, have at that stage was the totally impenetrable body armour that would permit me to sail through all the impending troubled waters of development without any resultant serious injury. So thank goodness for nicotine, alcohol and unrestricted access to powerful narcotics and long-acting tranquillizers.

Before the new surgery could be built I had to circumnavigate a process of delicate negotiation with the health authority with regard to the final layout: the number of rooms and their dimensions, for example, the overall size of the premises, access for the disabled and, most critically of all, where to locate the heated swimming pool with integral bar. As a soon to be single-handed GP I was also allowed an attached flat for a 'caretaker' to occupy.

This of course was in the dim and distant, dinosaur-like pre-mobile phone era, although having said that there remains even now a significantly large proportion of the practice area without any satellite coverage. I have since sent a text message to a friend in England from the Kosovo/Albanian border, but try and get the surgery to ring me when I am but a hundred yards down the road? Not a chance of it.

Somebody, therefore, had to be on hand in my absence to take messages, repel the bailiffs and know how and where to contact me at all times.

It would have to be someone in whom I had the utmost trust, and at this early stage I had no one in mind, but later, just when I needed her, cameth the hour, cameth the woman.

The advent of Evelyn . . .

She was running a farm with her son out in Coryton, one of the more rural areas of the practise some eight or nine miles distant from the surgery. Her husband had died suddenly a few years earlier, sadly uninsured, and his sisters – who were joint partners – had taken their share of the money and run, leaving mother and son to struggle on unsupported, often beyond the point of exhaustion.

The inevitable finally happened. Farming was hitting one of its many terminal downslides, and after a bad year with the lambs they could struggle no more. The farm had to go, and with it their home, their security and the last of their money. All future prospect of independence disappeared at a stroke, or so it seemed.

Although latterly a farmer's wife Evelyn had in her youth been a nanny. She was just made for the task, a natural, and had, I later learned, been born and bred in Lifton itself.

It was just so easy.

Empty flat above the surgery . . . homeless Evelyn . . . they were made for each other.

For years to come she was caretaker, friend, confidante and part-time mother to us all, and whenever a spare moment came her way she filled it with children. After so many years of struggling she had, I like to think, found a little bit of peace at last.

Although I initially intended to work single-handed, it remained my pronounced intention to take on a partner once I had built up the list size to sufficient proportions. The health authority might have been happy for Margaret to take me on as a very much junior partner in terms of both status and financial remuneration – as, come to think of it, so was she – whilst being groomed (I use the word loosely) to take over on her retirement, but the practice was too small in numbers to support two full-time younger GPs.

The provisional building plans seemed to be vast, but common sense – yes, a commodity you might be forgiven at this point for thinking I was genetically deficient in – dictated I incorporate as great a spare capacity as I could for the future. It was a more prescient decision than I gave myself credit for at the time, as now over fifteen years and one extension later, we are still looking for room to expand . . . as is the local cemetery.

Building the surgery was well beyond any of the nightmare scenarios I had envisaged. Despite having been in the vice-like grip – sorry, warm, encompassing embrace – of the NHS for less than a year, I could scarcely find my way around the myriad of winding country lanes leading off at unexpected tangents from Lifton, let alone the interminably indecipherable red tape of health authority bureaucracy.

I had firstly to arrange the financial backing, secondly hire the professional services of an architect – although I had then subsequently to disengage him two-thirds of the way through the project to seek an alternative, who might hopefully have some more cogent idea what it was he was supposed to be doing – and thirdly contract a builder with more sense than money, an almost impossible undertaking given the rocketing land prices at the time.

The architect and I each knew what we wanted, in terms of layout, design and the ability to price the whole enterprise according to our somewhat disparate wishes. My needs were essentially functional – a completed project within the time limits and budget available, and all constructed with regard to a few basic rules: i.e. he did what I said, when I wanted him to, and I would pay for it later. His self-determined remit, however, appeared to be diametrically opposed to my own, involving ubiquitous exterior wooden cladding, no less, the first of a series of Scandinavian lookalike constructions in the south-west.

'But I'm paying you,' I would remind him pointedly, 'and not the other way round.'

The critical moment, however, arrived one day when I asked him well into the latter stages of construction, 'So where is the sewage going to go, then? Because we will undoubtedly generate some . . .'

'To the mains drainage,' he replied dismissively, with an 'And how stupid are you?' look on his face.

'Ah, the mains,' I said icily. 'Would that be the same mains drainage which runs under the road passing the front of the surgery?'

'It would,' he agreed, with a sigh obviously intended to delineate my complete lack of comprehension of the technicalities involved.

'No,' I said, shaking my head sadly. 'I don't think so. Sewage generally runs downhill, and that . . . ' pointing in a northerly direction like a kindergarten teacher to an unruly pupil still uncertain of the direction of the toilets, ' . . . is undoubtedly up. Are we expecting our sewage to magically defy the forces of gravity? Or how, to put it in words of one syllable, do you imagine it might get from down here, to up there, without demolishing half the building and ripping up the access road to the car park? Looking around me I have yet to discover an army of willing volunteers who will carry it, one bucket-load at a time, from down here to up there on a regular basis. Or have you maybe just miscalculated, a touch? You are an architect, aren't you . . ?' I continued, as he paled visibly. 'At least, I had been reliably informed that you are, but I am now beginning to wonder . . . '

Have you ever noticed how lean, wiry, red-headed men begin to sweat profusely when put under pressure?

'Then we'll go the other way,' he suggested hastily. 'Down through the back, across that field behind the car park and out to the system on the main road in the village. That should . . . '

' . . . have been thought of an awful lot earlier,' I finished for him through gritted teeth. 'The laws of gravity do not to my knowledge appear to have altered fundamentally since the unfortunate day I employed you. And that field,' I continued pointedly, 'is not actually *my* field. It is somebody else's field. Do I need to explain precisely what that means?'

I probably didn't, in all honesty – but I went ahead anyway, and at some considerably pleasurable length, depth and volume. It cost me, in the end, a visit to the rightful owner of the field and the blank cheque I took with me, but nicely sweetening the blow was the fact that it cost the architect a whole lot more. Like, for example, the remainder of his contract with me.

The final negotiating point with regard to planning the overall design of the building revolved around the provision of a third consulting room. Yes, I know there was only one of me at the time, but I was well aware that the requirement would undoubtedly be there some years down the line.

'Well,' considered Mr Dawlish, the very helpful man from the health authority – his wife had just given birth to their first child, and I think he would have granted me anything I wanted, no matter how outlandish – 'you could have an additional facility here if you had a GP trainee in the practice.'

'But I don't,' I pointed out kindly. 'And I'm not qualified to be a GP trainer, even if I wanted to be one – which I don't think I do.'

'Ah, but you could go on a course,' he suggested persuasively. 'They run them in places like Exeter every six months. You could become a trainer without actually having to resort to employing a trainee . . . that would do it, for the purposes you need.'

It was an attractive prospect, but . . .

'I don't have the time,' I admitted sadly. 'There's so much to be done here as it is.'

He looked at me steadily and raised his eyebrows.

'Did I say now?' he asked rhetorically, 'or even in the next six months? I don't think so.'

'Something in blue,' I mused reflectively, 'I think something in blue for your baby.'

'You've got a year,' he responded dreamily, showing me his entire collection of family photographs, 'from the day you move into the completed building.'

The new surgery opened its doors on 1 July 1991. Fifty-one weeks later I was on my way to Exeter.

For most of the past year I had worked each and every day, and been on call every night and every weekend. Margaret had helped out when she could, but her enthusiasm was understandably waning, along with her health. I was exhausted, and in need of a break.

I drove up the motorway on a knife-edge. I had by now two children – Charlie, aged three, and Cressie (Cressida) now eighteen months – whom I adored but barely knew: they were often still asleep when I left the house in the morning and back in bed again when I came home. I had a (now ex-) wife who on a good day did much the same.

Strange things happen when you are alone, unhappy and away from home – or at least, I was hoping they would. This, for me, was decision time – an opportunity to take stock, a chance to reflect.

A week when I could drink loads, without worrying . . .

I had heard about the Exeter course well in advance, and from a variety of sources – none of which were particularly flattering.

'They split you up into small groups and make you cry a lot,' I was reliably informed.

'Not me they won't,' I promised. 'I don't do lachrymose. And besides – what for?'

Sunday evening, and I duly arrived at the hotel where we were based, making my way up to my room. Immediately outside my window was a spectacular view of the unquestionably beautiful Exeter Cathedral.

'Yes, I can be happy here,' I thought quietly, considering my options. Dinner? An evening walk through the rain-splashed streets, or a little preliminary reading for the forthcoming week? With the benefit of hindsight . . .

I went to the bar, and stayed there.

For the next couple of hours strangely familiar figures readily identifiable as fellow victims came, ate, and mysteriously drifted away. I heeded them not, and why should I? By the second pint I was visibly relaxing; by the fourth, all my cares and concerns were floating gently over an unheralded horizon, and by the sixth I was beyond any form of meaningful intellectual dialogue.

When I was half-way through my eighth, they sent someone to find me . . .

'Dr Sparrow?' said a bespectacled, earnest-featured chap, leaning horizontally over the table next to me. 'Dr Michael Sparrow?'

I nodded cautiously, in case the room should start to spin again.

'We've been waiting for you upstairs,' he explained with an oily grin.

'Well, that's awfully kind of you,' I acknowledged graciously, 'but I'm not really ready to go to bed yet, thanks, and when I am I think I can probably still just about make it on my own.'

'No, no, you don't understand,' he said, giving an uncertain little laugh. 'We've been waiting for you to join us in the evening session.'

'The evening session,' I said blankly. 'And which evening session might that be?'

'The evening session that is clearly mentioned in the introductory documentation which appears to be on the table in front of you,' he replied, hopping from one foot to the other in an agitated fashion. 'Which, by the look of it, you have obviously yet to read.'

'Oh,' I said meekly, '*that* introductory documentation. Best follow you up, then.'

In a small, first-floor ante-room to one side of the hotel I was belatedly absorbed in the warm, all-encompassing embrace of my 'group'. There were, altogether, seventy or so GPs and nurses on the course, randomly split into clusters of eight or nine jolly individuals in whose company we were to spend the bulk of the ensuing week. The all-important allocation process had taken place during my solitary but thoroughly enjoyable sojourn in the bar, and each group was now apparently fully embarked upon the 'getting to know you' process so essential to such occasions under the watchful eye of a series of tutors.

I took my seat with a sinking heart. Lawrence, our tutor, metaphorically embraced me as if I were the prodigal son returning from half a lifetime of self-imposed exile in the wilderness.

'Welcome, Michael,' he said, oozing insincerity from behind his expansive smile, 'to our group. We are so pleased you have managed to join us. Aren't we, everybody?'

'Oh yes,' they chorused enthusiastically, before I had any chance to respond. 'So pleased, yes, so very pleased to have you with us.'

'Really?' I murmured sarcastically, being just a tiny bit unimpressed.

'We've been playing a game,' continued Lawrence unctuously.

'Oh goody, I like games,' I said, interrupting deliberately. Get them on the back foot from the outset, that's my credo. 'Ludo? Darts? Or maybe rounders – I especially like rounders.'

'The name game,' said Lawrence, ignoring my second 'Really?' with a queasy smile. 'We've been throwing balls to each other . . .'

'Really?' I found myself saying again.

' . . . so as to become fully acquainted with each other's names and explore our developing personalities,' he persisted doggedly, beginning to sweat. 'It's one of the most crucially formative elements of the mutually enjoyable and self-determined reward-based bonding process we so trust you will want to share in. Over the next week we aim to become your friends, your family, your intimate confidants . . . We will by then be hopefully functioning as an interdependent team, a self-supporting, exclusively retrospectively seeking yet mutually symbiotic cell of empathic blood brothers, sisters and those with real and significant gender identity crises. Individuals who will care for you when you are down, rejoice with you during your brief but ecstatically transient periods of elevation, encompass your pain, your unexpurgated self-flagellatory instincts and take pleasure in the manifest expressions of your all too illusionary episodes of normality. It's what we are all about, it's what makes us feel so wanted and valued amongst our compatriots, it's . . . '

It's making me want to throw up, I wanted to say, but thankfully chose not to, being too overcome by a warm encompassing bout of nausea that might just possibly have been down to an over-indulgence of alcohol – combined with a criminally negligent lack of carbohydrate intake – to respond in a more adultly orientated focus group kind of way.

'So join us, do,' continued Lawrence joyously, changing tack hurriedly as he caught the look of potentially vicious retribution on my face. 'Watch us for a while as we throw the ball, or . . . ' he gave a little tinkling laugh at this point that made me want to vomit uncontrollably, ' . . . the spherical communicator, as we like to call it, around the circle, and each time you are unquestionably blessed by receiving it you are wonderfully empowered to tell us a little about yourself, and what qualities, what compassionately contributory offerings you would wish to bring to the group. I will now start again, to give you the general idea. The Spherical Communicator, Sarah, if you please.'

You had to admire the guy. But at the same time you had to wish upon him a lack of anal sphincter control in the most embarrassing of circumstances . . . The comically dysfunctional charade continued, unabated.

'I'm Lawrence,' he began, on receipt of the spher . . . well, the ball, actually, 'and I'm a GP principal, a GP lecturer and tutor in Exeter, and I am . . . ' he spread his arms expansively, ' . . . your leader, and count myself privileged to be so. I bring to the group my experience, my love of all my fellow men – and women, children and ethnically challenged asylum-seeking potential terrorists,' he added hastily, should any of them have been mortally offended, 'and add to that my sincere desire to get to know you all as soul mates, as well as colleagues, in the next few days.'

He tossed the ball across the circle of chairs to a thin, dark-haired woman immediately to my left.

'I'm Jackie,' she said, a disturbingly enthusiastic gleam of zeal in her eyes. 'I'm a practice nurse in Colchester, and I welcome the chance to bring to the group my love of humanity and my excitement, yes . . .'

Had I not known better, I would have sworn she was currently in the throes of some form of prohibited sexual ecstasy.

' . . . my excitement and anticipation that as a group we can overcome the formidable odds we all share as we reach into each other's hearts and souls and draw out the very depths of emotional commitment that will so sustain us into our interpersonal development-mental pre-programmed assignments. She turned towards me, and I blanched.

'I would like to welcome Mike into our amniotic midst as a valued member of the community, in the hope that he will rapidly come to share the common bond we have all so quickly begun to develop.'

She threw the ball across the divide to Tom, another GP from Exeter, as I tried to contend with the rising surge of bile in my throat threatening shortly to announce itself on the floral carpet. Round and round the circle it went, as one by one each partici-pant spoke volubly of their desire for world peace, an end to all famine and better discount schemes at the local supermarkets.

Only Malcolm, an engaging Scot with a wry sense of humour, seemed to be on my wavelength. Finally the ball found its unerring way back to Lawrence, who beamed at me with such a terrifying degree of 'lurve' in his heart that I thought for one glorious moment his eyes might pop out unexpectedly all over his curiously stained trousers.

'We have each,' he intoned sanctimoniously, 'opened our hearts, our inner feelings, and laid bare some of our inadequacies

201

. . . ' The guy was unstoppable, and had so many more to declare.
' . . . for all to see. We have each plumbed the depths, the dark,
impenetrable depths where Boy Scouts may roam nakedly
unencumbered by convention, where Madonna-like figures rise
seductively available yet unresponsive above us as we wallow
vaingloriously in the submerged trenches of our self-imposed
depravity, but now we have reached the promised land, a deserted
oasis of vermin-free, dolphin-rich, golden-sanded, palm-tree-
inhabited quays, an idyllic time tunnel of content where we can
all reinforce, we can all resubstantiate, where we can all
encapsulate those frailties within our inner souls and explore
them together and at last . . . '

I was transfixed. Lawrence tossed the ball to me and I caught
it, regarded it thoughtfully for a moment and then threw it
adroitly out of the open window into the street below.

'My name's Mike,' I said steadily, 'and this is all bollocks.
I'm an individual, not some zombified member of a group, and
I intend to remain that way. Forgive me for mentioning it but I
thought I was here for a week's instruction on how to become a
GP trainer, not to wallow in mutual declarations of love and
touchy-feely sentimentality. I don't have any particular need to
touch any of you right now, and I bloody well don't want any of
you feeling me, thank you very much. If I bring anything to the
group it will probably be my hangover in the morning. And
now,' as I stood up to leave in absolute, stunned silence, 'if you
will excuse me . . . '

'Nice going, Mike,' said Malcolm with a grin as he joined
me in the bar an hour or so later. 'They are now all discussing
how best to adjust to their feelings of rejection in the face of
your marginally unfavourable acceptance speech. Fancy a pint?'

It was a strange week.

Whilst, as far as I am concerned, group work and all that
bonding together stuff is, as I like to feel I put it so graciously,

complete bollocks, it made fascinating viewing for the interested observer. It was a people watchers' paradise – rather like *Big Brother* but without the cameras, nudity or intellectual conversation.

The following day I endeavoured to be a little more sociable – I'm not at all sure anyone noticed, but I tried all the same. The trouble was that no matter how hard I attempted to appreciate the finer points of the course, and glean some understanding of how it would assist me in my future career as a potential GP trainer, I failed completely. Gazing collectively into the depths of one's own – and then each other's – navel has never been my style, and strikes me as being wholly unproductive.

I was, however, strangely – almost worryingly – drawn to the entertainment value of grown men and women behaving like pre-pubescent children at a bun fight. If it was at times uncomfortably and unnecessarily intrusive it was at others compelling entertainment as each would launch headlong into their own personal catharsis, unravelling their psychological make-up for all to see in the fashion of a couple of kittens running amok in the dining room with a loosely bound ball of wool.

An interesting phenomenon took place midway through the third morning. There must have been a hell of a lot of undercover bonding going on in the previous two days because when, in their wisdom, the tutors decided to temporarily disband all the groups and restructure them for the final two sessions before lunch, there followed the captivating spectacle of unreconstructed mourning amongst the participants.

These, I had to remind myself, were professional colleagues; people occupying positions of responsibility and authority in their local communities; people in whose hands the lives and well-being of thousands of patients rested; people who were currently sulking petulantly in the corners of the room, throwing tantrums in the corridors and in several cases reduced to tears . . .

'They split you up into small groups and everyone cries a lot,'

I had been judiciously warned. And do you know what? Just about everyone did – apart from Malcolm and myself, that is.

We had taken to having an evening drink together, most of the rest of the course being given to early retirement to bed, no doubt exhausted after a day full of emotional outpourings. Malcolm, though no more given to lachrymose declarations of inadequacy or revelations of childhood enuresis than myself, was an altogether more pro-active participant in group sessions.

Several years younger than I, he had achieved in many respects so much more than I have even now, or probably ever will do.

'I had never realized,' he reflected towards the end of the week, 'how driven I was by the achievements of my older brother . . .' (a high-flyer in the medical world) ' . . . and how so much of what I've done has been to emulate his example.'

But he didn't cry as he said it, nor swallow hard and look misty-eyed into the distance – which is just as well or I would probably have throttled him on the spot.

As the week progressed I began at times to feel uncomfortable with some of the events I was witnessing. The tutors swapped around at regular intervals, and there seemed to me to be a shared, almost disturbingly voyeuristic quality about some of the sessions they ran. Maybe I do them a great disservice but it seemed at times as if they were quietly revelling in the distress it appeared they almost deliberately induced in their charges.

'Got him,' I could imagine them secretly rejoicing, mentally ticking off the appropriate box as another GP finally succumbed, sobbing heartbrokenly into their Filofax. But perhaps they were genuine in their motives, and I just a disenchanted cynic. Perhaps, on the other hand, West Ham will win the Premier League this year by a record number of points; perhaps the Tooth Fairy is real after all, and perhaps, just perhaps, I can give up smoking for a whole week without cheating . . .

On the fourth day, after a late night bout in the bar the evening before, I turned up three-quarters of an hour late to the first session of the morning. I raised my hand in apology as I entered the tutorial room.

'Sorry,' I shrugged, casually unrepentant. 'Overslept a bit – tiring, don't you find, all this wailing and gnashing of teeth?'

I was met, to my astonishment, by a sea of hurt and confused faces.

'We felt we couldn't start without you,' said Poppy, a short, dumpy woman who had been duly inaugurated as our final tutor the afternoon before. 'The group wasn't complete without you – we all thought that, didn't we, everyone?'

Everyone nodded dolefully.

'Yeah, right,' I began scathingly, 'of course you . . . '

'Of course you did!' I intended to finish, no doubt then indulging in some unnecessarily fulminating invective, which would have inevitably reinforced my perceived right to occupy the entirety of the moral high ground as it was currently available. But then I took another look around.

There were genuine tears in a couple of pairs of eyes, and Poppy – with whom I had yet to share all the electrically attractive affinity crackling between Little Red Riding Hood and the wolf – seemed unaccountably upset. Malcolm, in a chair set back slightly out of view from the rest, raised a gently restraining finger to his lips.

'Of course,' I repeated, suddenly and irrationally full of recalcitrance, 'of course you must have done. I'm so sorry . . . .'

And so it all went on.

Too many gut-wrenching tears, too little laughter, so much despair . . . not to mention a whole host of 'How do you feel/ what do you think you have been able to contribute to the course and the group?' type of questions in rapid succession from Poppy, Nigel, Lawrence or most sinisterly of all Godfrey, a man who resembled every photofit picture of a child-molesting, bank-robbing malcontent I have ever seen.

They were all disconcertingly interchangeable, spouting the

same religiously preconditioned protocols like some watered-down version of Robo-Cop, but without his innate sense of understated humour – and none of his awesome weaponry. It was all too much to be bearable.

It was our last night, and the obligatory valedictory dinner.

We travelled by coach to one of the local restaurants, gathered at a small reception in our honour to order preliminary refreshments and then watched in astonishment as everyone scuttled to the four corners of the room leaving Malcolm, myself, Lawrence and Godfrey in splendid isolation at the bar.

'Take a look around you,' said Lawrence, who had by now grudgingly accepted me as a fellow member of the human race, albeit one he wouldn't choose to hug a tree with. 'In all the time we have been running these courses I have never seen that before.'

The entire party had split up into their respective groups, tutors in tow, as they huddled secretively together in compact circles around their drinks, with not an intruder in sight.

'So tell me, Lawrence,' I asked curiously, 'and for once this is a genuine enquiry, not one of my usual side swipes at the establishment. Does this . . . ' he followed my gaze as it swept around the bar, ' . . . represent a successful culmination of your methods here, developing this quite remarkable interdependence amongst a collection of previously disparate strangers whose only common link is the profession they share? Or not? Over the last few days I've seen, you've seen – in fact we've all seen – people breaking their hearts in front of us over past and present personal crises, to be comforted by comparative strangers who tomorrow afternoon will return to their respective bolt holes all over the country. There have been more collective tears here than at the Wailing Wall in the course of a lifetime.'

I had never in fact visited the Wailing Wall at this point, but I have now, and was transfixed by the spectacle. The women, by and large, were wailing away with traditional gusto but the men, who looked very smart in their long black coats and hats, were all wandering around talking animatedly on their mobile phones, chain-smoking furiously.

Lawrence looked around the bar, deep in thought.

'Can you honestly say to me that this is true friendship?' I continued, unabated. 'What I see everywhere around me is casual acquaintanceship gone mad, under the most demanding of circumstances. Are we any of us the better for it – better GPs, better potential trainers, better human beings? And when any one of us wakes up on Sunday morning, supposedly safely back in our home environment, to confront a single one of the demons you have all but deliberately unleashed here, who will be there to rush to our aid? Who will come forward in our defence? Is that what you wanted, Lawrence . . ? Is that what you hoped to achieve? Is that what it is all about?'

Lawrence took a deep breath, sucking in the smoke-filled air as if it were some sort of lifeline, and looked across to Godfrey, then Malcolm, and back to myself.

'I don't think I know, any longer, Mike,' he said simply. 'For the first time since we've been doing this, I'm really not sure . . .'

We eventually returned, as one always does on such occasions, to the bar back at the hotel, and at last the various individuals in the hitherto stringently separated groups began to intermingle. All except one . . .

I sat on a stool by the bar watching, thinking, and trying to rationalize all that had passed. I had come away for a break, a chance to reconsider the future. The life I had at home was not the one I wanted, and tomorrow I had promised myself I would return with some decisions made, some concrete plans of action.

Failed there then, I thought wryly, raising a glass to myself and reaching for another cigarette. But then . . .

'I've been watching you all week,' said a soft, warm voice to

207

my left, which I hoped fervently wasn't that of the barman. As I turned to look around there she sat; Vicki – small, pretty, petite, with bobbed fair hair and a seductive Irish lilt to her voice. I don't think I had spoken a word to her in all the time we had been on the course.

'Why is it,' she continued, regarding me quizzically, 'that whenever everyone else is over there, you're over here by yourself, quite content in your own company? And yet if they were all to come over here I'd probably soon find you sitting alone over there. Why is that, Mike? It is Mike, isn't it . . ?'

'This morning,' said Poppy sombrely, 'we shall spend reflecting upon what we have achieved – '

'And then break for coffee in a couple of minutes?' I suggested brightly.

'Even at the very end,' she sighed with mock sadness, 'you still don't know when to keep quiet, do you? We shall, I hope, digest the various lessons we have learned, and discuss how we can take it all back to our homes and practices in a progressive, forward-looking way as better, more self-aware practitioners of our trade. I want you to grow in our reflected wisdom, take nourishment from our unconditional offerings and find succour in our frailties and honesty . . . '

'Right, done that,' I said briskly, after a second or two's thought. 'Can I go home now?'

The atmosphere was beginning to change.

'Thank you, Mike,' said Poppy, 'for your usual timely and deeply insightful contribution. Now please will you shut up, sit down, and listen to the rest of us . . . '

'Yet again,' said Malcolm, suppressing a grin.

I suppose it wasn't so bad, in the end. After lunch we drifted out into the garden.

'I want you,' Poppy had told us, actually smiling broadly for once, 'to spend a few minutes with each group. I want you to reflect together on what you have gained from each other's company, what you have learned of them and from them, but most of all what you have learned about yourself. Open your hearts, welcome the thoughts from the very depths of your innermost beings . . . '

I opened my mouth to speak, but she was there before me.

' . . . yes, I know it will be difficult for you, Mike, but hey, what the hell – why don't you give it a go? Stand back and consider what you will take home from the course – there have, I know, been criticisms in some quarters of what we set out to achieve . . . '

'I could offer a few more,' I said helpfully.

' . . . but happily you are not currently in control of our budget,' she continued smoothly, shooting a darkly humorous look in my direction. The girl was learning. 'However, whatever you might think of us and the methods we follow it is because we genuinely think it is right to challenge you in this way. If, as we have all sometimes seen over the past week, you are not in control of your own life, then how can you expect to be in control of anyone else's?'

I swallowed hard, feeling suddenly vulnerable. That, for an uncomfortable moment, had struck a chord, in a place I didn't want to recognize.

'So time to reassess our lives,' continued Poppy finally. 'Imagine you are shopping with each other at a supermarket; take away in your trolley whatever it is that you want, and leave behind on the shelves that which you have no need of . . . '

I wandered slowly round the garden with the rest of them, mouthing platitudes in turn at each passing face. As chance would have it, Malcolm and I were last to meet.

'Thanks, Mike,' he said simply, holding out his hand. 'It's been fun, hasn't it?'

'Yes,' I agreed, grasping it firmly, 'I do believe it has.'

'And if you ever come to Glasgow,' he continued . . .

'Which I won't,' I promised faithfully.

' . . . then I'll be out,' he confirmed solemnly, 'until you go home again.'

And Poppy?

'I've enjoyed your sense of humour,' she admitted reflectively, 'but I've hated the way you've made both me and some of the other tutors feel uncomfortable about ourselves and what we've been trying to do here.'

'Which is partly what I meant you to do,' I said honestly. 'So not everyone will agree with me, but if you want to know what I think . . . which you don't, really, do you? But I'm going to subject you to it anyway . . . then it's that you all live and work here, sheltering behind your facades of false sincerity and your shallow illusions of power whilst you feed off the weaknesses and failings of the poor buggers who pass before you. It's like some sort of morale-boosting emotional scaffolding, bolstering your crumbling egos as you bear flawed witness to the inadequacies of others. It might make you feel better about yourselves, but it is always at the expense of the dignity of others and you know what? – I've never felt the need for a certificate in moral bankruptcy. It's like being on the *Titanic* – you've carefully constructed what you think is this great unsinkable vessel but as soon as you get a leak beneath the waterline . . . your heads are barely above the rising tide, you're drowning, Poppy, I'm sorry to have to say it but you are, and it won't take a tidal wave for the rest of them to drown with you . . .'

I left the gardens deep in thought, to move on. But there was something I had to do first, something important . . .

I found her, in the end, waiting for me on a seat in the car park, tears welling in her eyes. We drove down to the river together, neither of us knowing what we should say.

'I don't want to go home, Mike,' she said finally, breaking the silence between us as she kicked her feet distractedly in the water. 'I have to, I know – I have a husband there, and children, and responsibilities. But I don't want to go home.'

'Neither do I,' I admitted, sitting down beside her.

We had sat and talked until dawn was almost upon us, at first in the bar and then – as the crowd dwindled around us – in her room, after leaving separately. Ironically it turned out that she was down at the end of the landing, immediately next to my room, and yet for five days we had not met, either leaving or going in. For five days, not even a chance encounter in the corridor . . .

It is so hard, and yet so easy, looking back after all these years, to recall how I then felt. For what turned out to be little more than a twelve-hour period, just half a day, I felt like I was inhabiting another world, a different existence in some parallel universe with the grim reality of life at home so many light years away.

We were both unhappy, both stuck in a rut we had previously thought too deep to escape from and both, if I am honest, looking for some sign, some catalyst to show that somewhere ahead was a way out.

We said our final goodbyes and travelled down towards the motorway, one behind the other, stopping on the slip-road for a moment or two, neither of us wanting to leave. And then she set off eastwards, and I west, back to the lives from which we had so briefly escaped.

We never met again.

It was, as so many things are in life, just never meant to be. I forget the quote, right now, about ships and their passing in the night, but for a while I often used to wonder . . . Had we met by chance outside our respective rooms on the first night, and not the last . . . Had we met so many years earlier, or maybe later, when our children were grown . . . Had we never met at all . . . where, under those circumstances, might I now be?

I look back as I write this, now nearly eleven years later and as happy as I could ever wish to be, with an air of quiet reflection. Of Vicki – I have no idea, but I hope, wherever she may be and whatever she may now be doing, that she will have like me found what we were both then looking for, all that time ago.

If she should read this one day – and I know you will know who you are – I ask only three things.

Remember that so very short time we both shared together; move ever onwards, if you can, to a better and more fulfilling life; and please could I have back the fiver I lent you for some petrol.

Whatever my opinion of the course, I knew when I returned home that something in my life had to change. The stresses we all face are generally so carefully hidden, from our patients and – more importantly – sometimes ourselves. Some doctors resort to drink, or drugs, in an effort to survive, and for others of us it is our marriage that has to give way, with all the heartache it involves.

If I could go back, I sometimes ask myself, to the isolation of that metaphorically uninhabited island in time, would I still choose to? And am I glad I was once there, albeit against any better personal instincts I once used to possess?

The answers have to be respectively 'No,' and then 'Yes', conclusively 'Yes', to the second.

We leave so many things behind us as we travel through life, so many memories, both the good and the bad. The trick, surely the trick to our long-term survival has to be to hang on to the good ones, remembering nostalgically how we felt at the time, and disregard the bad, and the sadness that must so often ensue.

We can leave it, in fact, on Poppy's supermarket shelf, from where it first came from – in a place we can always choose to visit, but no longer wish to go . . .

10

Finding my Feet

Back in the welcoming sanctuary of Lifton it was time to re-engage in that well-known, high-risk game of strategy and intrigue, namely, 'Getting to Know Your Patients Before They Get to Know You'.

I had still to master the preliminary bout of 'Getting to Find Your Way Around the Practice Area', but most woefully of all had failed the simple introductory test known locally as 'Leaving and Re-entering the Multi-Storey Car-Park Without Considerable Embarrassment'.

But then we all make mistakes.

My daughter, Cressie, at the tender age of four, had her own ideas about mine. She rested her chin in her hands and regarded me thoughtfully over the kitchen table.

'Being a doctor wasn't such a good idea, was it, Daddy?' she observed seriously.

Of course, it is not obligatory to be a doctor in order to make some *really* stupid blunders – it just helps. Anyone else could do it, were they to try hard enough, but mostly they don't have the advantage of the depth and breadth of our potentially humiliating circumstances. If you are unlucky enough to possess any form of medical qualification, then no matter how hard you may endeavour to disguise it, you may rest assured . . .

Stupidity will seek you out, if you can but wait long enough.

Shortly after my arrival in Lifton a multi-storey car park was built in the market square of the nearest town, Launceston –

though not, I have to report, without a great deal of heated debate. Feelings ran high – so high in fact that eggs were thrown at some of the local councillors, and after a few weeks I have to report that my right shoulder became sore . . .

I had never actually parked in the multi-storey car park, and on reflection I began to wonder why.

This was partly, I am ashamed to say, because I begrudged the fifty pence entry fee, but more realistically because I was never quite sure which bit you drove into and which bit you admired for its 'Dare to be different' architectural excesses. On the particular day in question I was left with no choice – all the double yellow lines throughout the rest of the town centre were taken, my disabled sticker was out of date, and I felt moved to be more adventurous than on previous occasions.

I drove into the car park – through the exit, I have to admit, but nobody seemed to notice – and planted Sheila, my 'You can get anything in a' Volvo across three spaces in what I kid myself was some sort of pathetic attempt at a protest. In reality it was probably no more than a parsimonious gesture – fifty pence a car, I calculated, means twenty-five pence a space if you park across just a couple of them, but by spreading your 'verging on a limousine' Volvo across an adjacent three . . .

16.6666p recurring per space. An absolute bargain.

Of course, no matter how hard you tried, you could only have parked my much loved but now sadly extinct Fiat Panda in one space at a time, which made it impossibly expensive to run.

So having left my car strewn untidily across the maximum number of available spaces, I looked haplessly around for the way out, which was by no means as simple a task as it might sound. Having failed completely to spot it within a dragonfly's lifespan I resolved to use my initiative, and followed the chap in front of me. It worked a treat – I descended a long flight of stairs, passed through a couple of swing doors and there I was, out in the street in the middle of the town. I thought I might manage to cope, from there.

I am generally not very good in towns – I tend to forget what I am doing there, unless I have a list, and more often than not I forget that I should have brought a list and spend my time window shopping in front of the banks, wondering idly which one of them is actually mine. You must know the feeling – one of you has my money, but I have no idea which one of you it is, or how I'm ever supposed to get it out.

I have not, I think, walked into a bank and withdrawn real money for some five or more years. Quite frankly the cashiers intimidate me.

Still, having for once successfully finished all my business in town I made my way back to the multi-storey. I decided to follow the same tactic for re-entry and simply followed the woman in front of me – in through a couple of swing doors, round a blind corner, through another door, and there I was.

The trouble is, there I was right in the middle of the ladies' loo. It would perhaps have mattered less had there not been three or four ladies also there, regarding me with expressions I hoped desperately were merely ones of curiosity and not recognition.

I think I was even more surprised than they were, so I took the only course of action available to me.

'It's OK,' I said as nonchalantly as circumstances would allow, 'I'm a doctor,' and I turned tail hurriedly and walked out.

Even finding my way to branch surgeries seemed to be fraught with difficulty, let alone dealing with what you might find there.

Branch surgeries tend these days to be the final reserve of us neolithically established rural communities, and our practice currently has four of them. They all take place in local village halls – although one of them is temporarily suspended, the venue having fallen foul of the fire regulations . . . it hadn't got any. It was no more than five years ago, however, that the one I most enjoyed visiting used to be held in the front room of an elderly patient's house.

The sick, the needy and those just wanting a cup of coffee and a sticky bun would gather together in the dining room with the elderly lady occupant (who rented the premises from another, even more elderly patient of mine) where they would enjoy a full and frank exchange of views on local issues – in other words, a jolly good gossip. Whenever I could prise any of them away I would then see them in the sitting room, possibly the most ill-equipped branch surgery in creation. You could just about take a patient's blood pressure, or on a good day – if the wind was in the right direction – maybe look in their ears, but anything even vaguely involving all those areas from the waist down that wasn't actually feet was completely beyond any form of rudimentary assessment.

This wonderfully alternative location is sadly no longer available to us, the owner of the house having died and the lady who rented it having moved on, subsequently dying herself. Unfortunately, as so often seems to happen in the country, there was a tiny misunderstanding as to the anticipated timescale of events, and the new owners moved in a week earlier than I had been given to understand.

Not surprisingly, I had some interesting explaining to do when they returned from their leisurely morning shopping expedition for a little light lunch and found me examining a particularly purulent varicose ulcer in their front lounge bay window.

We now see patients from this particular village in the village hall kitchen, despite the absence of such routine commodities as chairs or tables, let alone couches or curtains. But even this downbeat location is salubrious in the extreme compared to the branch surgery venue I visit on Mondays and Fridays. This, believe it or not, is held unceremoniously in another village hall, but this time in the loo.

In the ten years I have been doing this it has never once been decorated, although that is not to say it has been entirely ignored – somebody has removed both the table and chair I used to sit at and write on, for a start. Not content with that, the red plastic

couch beneath the coat rack has been refurbished with what looks
to be an old bit of curtain, which I am convinced is unquestionably dirtier – and, improbable though it may seem, even less
hygienic – than the original covering.

No longer are we able to bully the occasional patient to lie
down upon it, and I for one can't say I blame them.

We recently had Claire, a medical student from Bristol, stay
with us as part of her general practice training.

'Oh no, you don't,' she said firmly as I related to her the details
of the above branch surgery. 'You have to be joking . . . '

'Oh yes, you do,' she said faintly, half an hour later as a small
boy wandered between us and the elderly lady we were trying
to examine to have a pee in the loo just beside us, neglecting in
his urgency to bother to close the intervening door.

One day, they have promised, they will provide us with our
own room, and a door that actually closes. Just like one day when
I get to be Prime Minister I shall give out dolly mixtures on the
NHS and declare Devon and Cornwall an administrator-free
zone, enforcing within my first week of office their complete
and irrevocable exile to at least as far as Bristol.

Eighteen months into the job I was beginning at last to come
to terms with the vagaries of country life, and the wily ways of
some of our patients. You had, on occasion, to be even sneakier
than they were, which meant dispensing with every word you
could recall of the Hippocratic oath.

Of course, all doctors are honest – just like all Scotsmen are
generous, all Welshmen impartial, all Irishmen reserved with
strangers, and all Englishmen great fun at parties.

We always give our patients the complete, unabridged truth,
no matter what the circumstances, no matter how much pain
and suffering it may inflict upon . . . well, upon them, of course,
as opposed to ourselves. After all, who could possibly be hurt
by the uncomplicated honesty of, say, 'All right, Mr Elsworth,

if you really want to know I give you about a week and a half. I guess planning for your Golden Wedding is going to be pretty pointless – well, for you it is, anyway . . .'

We are all of us, during the course of our professional lives, faced with the occasional corns of a dilemma (my wife, on proof-reading this, wondered mildly if I actually meant horns, and probably I did. But I kind of like corns a bit better . . .).

Sylvia and Gerald Pengelly lived in an isolated tied cottage no more than a mile or so from the surgery. They had little in the way of the comforts of life – no gas, no public transport, no running water or indeed any form of indoor sanitation – but they did have their own well, together with an antiquated but still functioning pump, a tin bath and a grease-ridden Rayburn – a sort of old-fashioned precursor to the Aga, for the uninitiated.

And they had no near neighbours to turn to, nor had ever wanted them.

'We got our 'ealth, we got a few sheep an' 'ens, an' we got each uvver,' Sylvia would say contentedly. 'What more could we be possibly needin'?'

What more indeed?

'But you can't be all that comfortable,' I would argue. 'Think of it . . . there's Social Services who could help, for instance. I'm sure they could install one or two things that might make life a bit easier for you . . . an indoor toilet perhaps, and rails to help you get about. Double-glazing, maybe . . . ' moving into the realms of fantasy, ' . . . a dishwasher, satellite TV, a commode which still has its own lid on . . . '

'Yes, dear,' Sylvia would reply, 'I'm sure you've got all those things you need, an' I 'ope they make you very 'appy. But I was born 'ere, I've lived 'ere all my life, an' I reckon I shall die 'ere, so I will. You just see if I won't.'

'And so was I,' put in Gerald unexpectedly, given that I had thought he was fast asleep in front of the Rayburn, 'and so have I, and so will I,' he finished adamantly.

Yes, I know what you are thinking – both born there, both lived there all their lives, yet married to each other . . . Well, this is deepest, darkest Devon, you must remember. We try not to ask too many questions.

At the age of ninety-six, Sylvia lost her husband. I found him – following her frantic call to the surgery – beneath the bed, Gerald having successfully located the chamber pot for the first time in some years.

And at the age of ninety-seven, Sylvia acquired for herself a lodger . . .

But not just any lodger. Oh no, this was a mere toy boy, a slip of a lad, seventy-six years of age with a reputation and unhealthy aroma that went a long way before him. He had once allegedly threatened Dr Margaret with a shotgun – which marked him out as either a brave man, or an incredibly foolish one – and on another occasion had apparently tried to run her down in his Land Rover whilst she was out walking her terrier along the lane from the surgery.

But he missed. His eyesight was awful.

Doctors in general – and GPs in particular – sometimes have a difficult ethical position to contend with when it comes to assessing the fitness of our patients to drive. For a start, we have all been medical students, and most medical students of my past acquaintance were unfit to drive pretty much most of the time, for one reason or another – not that that necessarily stopped any of us.

Our problem – in the pre-breathalyser days – was generally one of unadulterated inebriation, though I have to say that if Sylvia's lodger had been routinely under the influence of alcohol when behind the wheel of his car it would probably have improved his roadworthiness no end.

He just could not see to drive.

To be honest, I don't think he could see to walk, half the time, or sit, or probably even crawl. But drive he did, and in a fashion all of his own. I followed him down the main road, once, as he was weaving from side to side of both lanes with no clear idea of where the grass verge was – or even a vague one, I suspect – until he bumped into it. I watched from a safe distance, transfixed, and it was only when I finally overtook him as he turned off inadvertently into the slate quarry, no doubt mistaking it for home, that I realized who the driver was.

'Oh, it's only old Jim,' I thought to myself in amusement, and then I caught myself suddenly. It might be only old Jim, but old Jim's car could kill somebody as easily as the next man's. It was certainly food for thought.

They had a curious relationship, lodger and lodgee, about which I would never have speculated had I not called in to visit one afternoon and found Sylvia and the tin bath in the kitchen, as usual.

Except that this time Sylvia was standing in it, stark naked and shivering, and Jim was emptying buckets of cold water over her head. Neither of them seemed half as perturbed by my presence as I was by theirs, so I mumbled something suitably incoherent and beat a hasty retreat.

Over the next few weeks Jim began to cause me a considerable problem or two, or at least, his inability to see where he was driving did. He was diabetic, so arthritic he could barely turn his neck more than a few degrees sideways, and had dense cataracts in each eye. As a result of the latter he wore glasses that I swear must have originally been intended for somebody else – probably Sylvia's late husband, if the truth be told. We do so like to share our limited resources in the country, except with the non-indigenous population.

But what was worse, I was convinced he had recently suffered a minor stroke, with quite possibly another one not so very far away round the corner.

It wasn't just that Jim couldn't see – that on its own might not have been quite so terrifying. It was more his unshakeable belief that it did not affect his driving in any way that was causing all the trouble.

He was now in possession of an aged, all but terminally rusted crimson A40, a vehicle I now think almost certainly extinct in today's society. It had – surprise, surprise – just the one or two dents in it, or to be more accurate there were just a couple of small unblemished areas of bodywork interspersed between his personal amendments to the original.

It wasn't even that he drove too fast, either, because he didn't. He drove so appallingly slowly you could still have overtaken him had you been at the wheel of a written-off combine harvester, probably in reverse gear whilst going uphill in a blizzard. And if this should at first sight seem totally far-fetched I can personally vouch for it, unassailably, because one of my patients actually managed it. Twice, in the same morning.

Jim's meandering from one side of the road to the other had to be seen to be believed, and I suppose there was a certain logic to his dogged persistence. He couldn't see how mind-numbingly dangerous he could be, so it probably never occurred to him to believe it – just as he couldn't see the white lines down the middle of the road. Or the kerbs. Or even any oncoming vehicles.

It was only after following his terrifyingly erratic progress along the thankfully uninhabited lanes near the surgery for the third time in the space of a week that I resolved at last to take some action. Letting his tyres down was an option, but one doomed to failure – he just wouldn't notice, I thought resignedly.

My staff were instructed on pain of death, therefore, to refuse him any repeat prescriptions until he came to see me. It always works a treat, this approach – especially with those suffering from constipation – and sure enough Jim duly arrived at the surgery less than a week later.

I studied him as he sat before me in my consulting room, filthy old cap resting on his equally filthy old knee. He was wearing a tweed jacket and a waistcoat that had no doubt once been clean and respectable, but only before he had bought it and taken it out of the shop. He, likewise, peered across the desk at me – or at least he peered across at where he thought from previous experience I probably would be – and said in his characteristic, 'Devon meets Dallas' drawl:

'Nah then, doctor. What's all this, then? Stopped all me tablets, 'ave you?'

'No, Jim,' I replied honestly. 'I just thought it was time I should give you a bit of a check over.'

'I'm getting on fine, doctor, thank you,' he said amiably, starting to rise. 'Will that be all, then?'

'No, Jim,' I said again, as firmly as I could. 'To tell you the truth, I'm a bit concerned about your eyesight . . .'

'My eyesight's fine, doctor, thank you . . .'

' . . . and the effect it's having upon your driving . . .'

'My driving is as good as ever, doctor, thank you for asking,' said Jim, standing up to leave once more. 'Can I have my tablets now then, now that we've had this little chat together?'

'No, Jim,' I said, beginning to feel that all too reminiscent well of frustration building up within me. There was a certain familiar rhythm developing to this consultation, and I had to grit my teeth and steel myself to carry on.

'The fact is, Jim,' I continued determinedly, taking a deep breath and counting silently to ten, 'that I have to check your eyesight and see if it is good enough for you to carry on driving.'

'Well, you tell anyone you need to it's just fine, doctor,' he said expansively, 'and I'll be thanking you for taking such an interest. And now I think I'll be off, if it's all the same to you.'

'No, Jim,' I snapped, 'I'm afraid it is *not* all the same to me, as a matter of fact. I have to physically check your eyesight by getting you to look at a chart and read some letters out for me.'

He stood up for the third time, in high dudgeon. 'Oh, I haven't got time for all that now, doctor, I've got some sheep that need seeing to' – Poor sheep, I thought – 'and an evening meal to prepare.' And poor Sylvia, I worried more pertinently.

'So some other time then,' continued Jim, as if we had just agreed to meet for a few drinks together. I sat speechless as he walked to the nearest door and opened it, disappearing briefly into the examination room. 'Maybe next year, doctor,' he announced, re-emerging completely unabashed a moment or two later and turning belatedly to the other door out to the waiting room. 'You just tell them I can see fine. That'll do it, all right.'

'No, Jim,' I exclaimed once more, completely exasperated, bounding across the short gap between us and putting my hand on his shoulder to stop his departure. 'I can't do that until I've proved it beyond all reasonable doubt . . . '

God, you sound like Perry Mason, I thought absent-mindedly.

' . . . that you are fit to drive. And if you won't voluntarily submit yourself to an eye test then, much though I hate to do it, I have to inform you that I will now consider you physically unfit until such time as you do so.'

Goodness, I can sound officious when I want to.

'Right-oh, doctor,' he said, completely unconcerned. 'I'll be off then, presently, and I'll thank you again for your time.'

I resisted the impulse to kick him firmly in the shins. 'But you do understand,' I warned him exasperatedly, 'that you can't drive until I've checked your eyesight properly?'

'Yes, doctor, thank you, if you say so.' A sly look slid across his face. 'But I've got to get my car home first, now haven't I? Can't leave it out there all day blocking up your drive.'

I groaned inwardly, and gave up. It wasn't so very far he had to go, and as it was the school holidays the roads were all but deserted.

'I suppose you must, yes, Jim,' I accepted. 'But only this once, mind, this is the very last time. Promise me you won't be driving the car again, will you, until I've given you the all-clear?'

'If you say so, doctor,' said Jim, just as if I'd said, 'Mind your head on the way out,' or 'Have a nice rest of the day, won't you?' 'I always like to take heed of your advice.'

Three days later he was back in the surgery, collecting Sylvia's routine monthly medication.

By sheer chance I was out at the front desk at the time, checking to see if my next patient had arrived, and saw him waiting by the dispensary hatch. But, more importantly, by dint of some unaccustomed prehistoric instinct I just happened to walk across to the rear window of the building only to see his battered old wreck of a car abandoned three parts of the way into the hedge at the far end of the surgery car park.

'So you drove here, then, Jim,' I said sternly, having made my way back.

'Yes, doctor,' he said ingenuously. 'How else would I be getting Sylvia's tablets safely back home to her, otherwise, and her so in need of them and all?'

'But *Jim*,' I exploded, 'I quite specifically told you *not* to drive until you've had your eyesight checked, and you've just gone and done it *again*. Did you not *listen* to what I was telling you? Now – if you can see them – watch my lips. Do not drive from this moment onwards, ever, until I say that you can. Got it?'

I waited whilst he considered this news in his customary unhurried fashion, and then passed judgement.

'Right-oh, doctor,' he said eventually. 'But I've still got to get the car home, and Sylvia's tablets, haven't I?'

A week later he was in the surgery once more, collecting his own prescription. I missed him on this occasion, but my receptionist rang through to me and said that she had seen him get into his car and drive off, narrowly missing a lamp-post.

'Oh no,' I sighed resignedly. 'Which one?'

'The one that blew down in the 1990 gales and you relocated in your back garden,' she confirmed, 'and that you can only get to via your conservatory . . .'

224

Had he hit it he would no doubt have subsequently sworn it had strayed inattentively into his path just when his attention was temporarily diverted, and was to be held totally to blame.

Incensed, I rushed out to my own car and drove the mile and a bit down to the house he shared with Sylvia. Jim was standing by his car as I arrived, having obviously just climbed out of it.

'Hello there, doctor,' he greeted me in his usual drawl, 'just getting my tablets out of the car. Must have left them in there last week, and only now remembered, so I have.'

'Jim,' I said, very slowly and deliberately, 'I know full well that you have just driven down to the surgery and back, in your car, completely against everything that I have told you. And not only that, told you – as you must undoubtedly well know – on a whole lot than more than one occasion.' I was building up a good head of steam here.

'Have I, doctor?' asked Jim, somehow managing to look genuinely surprised. 'I suppose I must have done, if you tell me I have, but I can't say I can remember having done so. Sorry about that, I am. I would have thought it was last week, really I would. Are you sure it was today, and not another?'

'You know damn well what day it is,' I spat out. 'This is your last warning, Jim. I won't tell you again.'

Without the least trace of sarcasm he doffed his cap and said, 'Thank you, doctor, for taking so much trouble with me. Wishing you a good morning, then,' and limped off arthritically through the gate into his and Sylvia's cluttered yard.

Two weeks later, and here we were all over again.

Jim was sitting before me in my consulting room, on this occasion for a blood test for which he had unusually attended on the right day of the right week. It was at completely the wrong time, of course, but at least it seemed transiently that things might be improving.

225

I took his blood without difficulty, and as he was rolling down his sleeve I said casually, 'Did you drive here this morning, Jim?'

He looked me squarely in the face and said, 'I don't believe I did, doctor, after listening to all you had to say to me. I don't believe I did.'

I clapped him on the shoulder delightedly.

'Good, Jim, I'm so pleased to hear it. Would you like me to test your eyesight now?'

'No need, doctor, thank you. I don't think it will be necessary, now I'm not driving no more.'

He ambled off happily through my surgery door, and I sat reflecting for a moment. Good old Jim – he had listened to me at last. It was quite unlike him, after all these years. In fact it was, on reflection, completely unlike him at all . . .

I sprang into action.

Slipping out of the back door of my consulting room I dashed across the surgery car park, sped round the corner and down the road and was sitting on the bonnet of Jim's car as he wheezed asthmatically into sight. He was completely unaware of my presence, at first, only finally realizing I was ahead of him when I stuck my leg out to one side, like a gate at a level crossing, and he walked right into it.

'So you didn't drive here then, Jim?' I said icily.

'Good Lord, doctor, are there two of you?' he responded, completely unfazed, 'and why are you sitting on somebody else's car?'

'I think it is actually your car, Jim,' I said, chillingly polite. 'Your car that you indisputably told me you hadn't driven here today. At least, I think that's what you said.'

Jim let out an explosion of such beautifully observed violent anger that even I was impressed, despite myself.

'Kids,' he expostulated, 'the bloody kids of today. The things they get up to. You leave your car at home, trusting it to be safe, and this is what happens. What is this world of ours coming to, doctor, I ask you? What indeed?'

'It's coming to a driving ban, Jim,' I said lightly, 'and it's heading your way.'

I slid easily off the bonnet of his car and sauntered away, whistling cheerfully. Got you, I thought, in a fleeting moment of triumph.

Except, of course, that I hadn't.

The rules of medicine are that you can tell a patient they are patently unfit to drive, and advise them that it is their legal duty to inform the DVLC of their state of health, but that is as far as it goes. They can, if they choose, continue to blithely ignore you, driving on for as long as they wish.

In nearly every case like this I have ever come across, the rules of patient confidentiality prevent you from doing a damn thing about it.

Until the catastrophe inevitably happens. Then – and you can all but guarantee it – the coroner will fix you with a gimlet eye at the inquest and say, 'But you knew he was unfit to drive, Dr Sparrow,' in an incredulous tone, 'and yet you did nothing about it?'

But Jim was so unsafe, and so dangerous to all concerned, that I swallowed the last vestiges of my ethical convictions. After a long and fruitful conversation with my professional defence union I picked up the phone and rang a friend of mine at the local police station.

'Look, John, but off the record, please,' I began. 'It's about one of my patients, a Mr Denton – Jim Denton, you probably know him, down the road from me in Lifton – and his driving. Basically he's just not fit to even open the door of his own car, let alone any other, and God preserve us all if he gets into the driving seat and turns the engine on. He frightens the willies out of me every time he gets the bloody thing moving, and I've told him that countless times. But he just keeps on driving anyway, and I'm terrified. The surgery is right next to the local primary school, and who knows how long it's going to be before he runs down one of the children there. You have to do something about his licence, John, before he kills somebody, or – '

'Stop burbling, Mike,' said John calmly, 'and give me a few details. Date of birth – no, his, you idiot, not yours – address, postcode and telephone number. I'll tap him into the computer and see what comes up.'

There was a silence at the other end of the phone for a few minutes, and then:

'Licence,' mused John thoughtfully, 'and which licence is that you were talking about? According to our records he's never even passed a driving test . . . '

A few months later I was called to see Sylvia, who had pneumonia and was seriously ill. For all that, she was still pottering around the house with some unexplained mission in mind, searching distractedly through all her drawers and cupboards whilst clutching a large, kitchen sink sort of handbag as if her very life depended on it. Every now and then she would glance to the left and right with overtly pantomime-like gestures before peering back inside the bag to recheck its contents.

When she saw me arrive she suddenly stopped, and sagged down on a chair by the scullery table as if the weight on her shoulders was just too much to bear.

'Ninety-eight years,' she said sadly, 'an' not once 'ave I spent a night out of my own 'ome. I suppose now you're goin' to 'ave to send me to 'ospital, dear, aren't you?'

It was inevitable. I examined her carefully, and with a heavy heart explained, 'I have to, Sylvia. I do understand how you feel, really I do, but I can't just leave you here, like this . . . ' I waved my hand round in a forlorn gesture. 'Not here, not like this. You need some special help and treatment, so much more than I can give you at home.'

She nodded slowly, in calm acceptance.

'I know, dear,' she said in resignation. 'I've just been saying goodbye to my 'ouse while I was waiting for you to come. Better way, I thought. I think I'll not be back again.'

She looked over her shoulder in conspiratorial fashion, beckoning towards me before saying in an elaborate stage whisper as she motioned surreptitiously towards Jim, 'You can't trust 'im, m'dear. 'E's just like all the rest of 'em, after me money – and I got a bit put by, you know,' she added secretively. 'None of 'em are sure where it is, or 'ow much I've got, but they know it's around 'ere somewhere . . .'

She stopped for a moment, coughing violently.

' . . . an' they all think it's theirs, each an' ev'ry one o' them, by rights,' she continued weakly, temporarily recovering her composure. 'I've got this bag 'ere, wot I've kept until this moment. Look after it for me, dear, if you will. I know I can trust you to do the right thing with it.'

She passed me her bag and I took it out to my car, locking it in the boot without further thought. She was just a little old lady, I mused, with her funny ideas, and now was not the time to disabuse her . . .

Sylvia, bless her, died less than four hours after arriving at hospital, before the night had set in. As I heard the news the next day I felt so awful for having sent her away from her home, at the end of her life. But later, driving home that night, I suddenly stopped the car and began to smile.

Sylvia had maintained her record, the one that was so important to her. She had never once in her life spent a night away from her home.

A couple of weeks later Sally, my receptionist, stuck her head apologetically round the door.

'You've got visitors,' she hissed, motioning over her shoulder. 'I think it's Cinderella's ugly sisters, before they've got around to putting on their make-up.'

I must have looked a touch vacant – a hitherto unknown occurrence at my surgery. Sally took the hint, and responded accordingly.

'Mrs Pengelly's nieces,' she explained. 'They make sulphuric acid look comparatively benign and harmless.'

They came into my office as if they were bailiffs and I was about to be repossessed. For a minute or two I thought there must be dozens of them, so much noise were they making, but when the grey mists cleared I realized there were just the two. One of them was impossibly thin, wrinkled and hatchet-faced, and the other – when I could bear to look at her – was even thinner, yet more wrinkled and indisputably more hatchet-faced than the first, if that were possible.

'We know she had money . . . ' hissed Sister Number One.

'We just know she did,' agreed Sister Number Two sibilantly. 'But we've looked everywhere and we can't find it.'

' . . . anywhere . . . ' continued Sister Number One.

'So we think *he* must have taken it,' said . . . well, you'll have got the picture by now, 'and we want you to *find* it for us.'

'Because you're his *doctor*,' said Sister Number One triumphantly – they talked a lot in italics, these women – 'and you can ask him what he *did* with it.'

'Because it's *ours*,' they chorused together.

I could not decide which one I liked less, on first impressions, or to put it another way which of them I despised more – they both had an equally compelling case to present. After a long and painful consultation I ushered them eventually out of the door, their voices still ringing in my ears.

'We're her only living relatives,' said Sister Number Two virtuously.

'And she *owes* us,' said Sister Number One. 'Looked after her *proper*, Nell, all these years. Didn't we just?'

They had names, I thought, surprised.

'We did *too*, Em,' said Nell sanctimoniously. 'None better.'

'Then how come,' I couldn't stop myself from saying, 'I've never met either of you in my time here to date, or on any of the times I have visited? I've never even *heard* of you. Where in God's name have you been for the past five years when you should have been looking after Sylvia? Getting the surveyors in to calculate your anticipated inheritance, perhaps? Planning how to convert their long-cherished home into upwardly mobile flats for up-country incomers? You know the sort – more money than sense and just longing to come down and experience the "real" West Country until some itinerant cow wakes them up at five in the morning, or a fox slaughters their hand-reared two lambs and one chicken.'

I was, I think it must be said, beginning to warm to my task.

'And I have to say,' I continued, 'that if the squalor I recall seeing in the past in that house was what you now call "looking after her proper", then I sincerely hope I shall never meet anyone you claim to have looked after badly. It's only in the last two years that it has been much better, and I know for a fact you haven't been there in all that time. Someone else must have been helping out, instead.'

I had the brief pleasure of seeing them momentarily taken aback, and resolved to take advantage of it.

'Good day,' I said, '*ladies*,' stressing the word deliberately and relishing the fact that to my surprise it actually shut them up for a few seconds. 'Close the door behind you, if you please.'

They left, bridling indignantly as I slumped back in my chair, breathing heavily and trying to recover from their mauling. A cup of coffee, a cigarette or two, a moment's reflection . . .

And then I sat bolt upright, gulping for air. Sylvia's handbag. I rushed out to my car, where it was still lying undisturbed in the boot . . .

Twenty minutes later I sat behind my desk, having counted the unexpectedly large amount of cash that lay before me. I thought of dear old Sylvia, and how I had last seen her.

231

'Look after it for me, dear,' she had said, shortly before she died. 'You've been my doctor for so many years. I know I can trust you to do the right thing . . . '

I thought of her nieces.

'It's ours,' they had hissed together viciously, 'and we want to know where it *is* . . . '

I had something in the region of £20,000 in used notes piled up in front of me on my desk. Not a single person in the village, the county, or possibly even the entire universe had any clue whatsoever as to their existence. I just sat and thought, for the rest of the night.

So what would you have done?

I am as honest, I hope, as the next man. I consulted my conscience, rehearsed my entry speech to the Pearly Gates – should I ever finally get there – and did the same as I am sure would have you.

So it is of course a complete coincidence that some three months later I changed my ageing Fiat Panda for a brand new, top of the range Volvo convertible, with a state of the art CD player and extra flip-up seats in the boot.

Isn't it?

Well, actually . . . yes, it is.

A week later I drove far out past Sylvia's former house and pulled up outside a modest, semi-detached residence in a glorious valley way beyond my practice boundaries. Two small girls were playing contentedly in the tiny front garden, and came running excitedly up to the gate as I drew to a halt.

'Have you brought us our new puppy?' shrieked the eldest, of maybe five. 'Oh goody, goody, goody . . . Mummy said we couldn't afford one. What's she called, can we call her Tilly, please, please, and is she all little and warm and cuddly?'

'I'm so sorry,' I replied gently, 'but I am not the puppy man – perhaps your mum can tell you about that later. But you can help me – is your mum in? Do you think I could talk to her?'

'Yes, I'm in,' came a soft, guarded voice from my right, emerging from behind the remnants of a broken-down garage. 'But might I ask who it is that is wanting to know?'

'You must be Stephanie,' I said. 'I have something for you.'

'I've got relatives,' Sylvia had told me, 'but they don't do nothing for me – don't come round or help me with cleanin' or meals and things like that. All they want is me 'ouse when I dies, an' I keeps tellin' 'em its rented . . . ' she gave me an exaggerated wink, following up conspiratorially, 'but it ain't rented at all. Me an' Johnny (her late husband) we bought it an' owns it an' always 'as done . . . but there ain't none of 'em as knows it. But there's this girl, I calls 'er me niece – she's married to a relative of a nephew of mine – wot comes around most days to see if I'm orlright. She takes care of me proper, does Steph, 'eart o' gold, and nuffing too much trouble – I want to take care of her too, when I've gone, but I don't suppose I'll be 'ere to sort of organize it.'

There were tears now running down her cheeks.

'I'm old, and I know that I'm dyin'. Would you take care of it for me, please? I'm too tired to sort it out now, but I know I can trust you to do wot I am asking. Promise me . . . '

'I was Sylvia's GP,' I told Steph, who looked at me initially as if I was an unwanted intruder into her quiet life. 'It was me that admitted her to hospital the night she died, but before she went in she gave me this for safe keeping and made me promise to give it to you in person. So now I've come to do it.'

'What's in it?' she asked warily, eyeing up the plastic bag.

'Call it a lifetime's supply of puppy food,' I said with a smile.

She took the bag, glanced in it and blanched, sitting down suddenly. 'Oh my goodness,' she said faintly, 'there must be . . . it looks like . . . how much is in here?'

'I haven't counted,' I answered honestly. 'I thought I might leave that pleasure to you.'

233

'But I can't take it . . . ' She was totally overcome, visibly shaking. 'She shouldn't have . . . It's not mine . . . '

'Point me to the kettle,' I suggested, 'or maybe the cooking sherry instead, and I'll tell you all about it.'

She was right out of cooking sherry, but she did have some rather delectable elderflower wine and for once I broke my unshakeable rule when at work of not drinking until lunchtime.

'I can't take it,' she repeated later, shaking her head. 'We weren't even related, not directly, she had two nieces . . . '

'I've met them,' I grimaced, 'just the once, but the memory still lingers. Look, Steph, Sylvia may have been old and dying but she had all her marbles about her and she knew what she wanted. She trusted me to carry out her final wish, and that is what I have every intention of doing. I couldn't live with myself if I let her down. Right now, this money is mine to do with what I think fit. I didn't have to come here – I could have handed it to the lawyers, her bank manager, the "ugly sisters", or invested in a new people carrier for myself with removable seats and an integral icemaker. No one would ever have known, apart from me – and probably Sylvia rotating in her grave until the crack of doom. Am I beginning to get this across to you?'

She nodded silently.

'It's yours, Steph,' I reiterated. 'I will swap it for another glass of elderflower wine. Is it a deal?'

Steph's two daughters, hovering on the fringes of the conversation, were hopping excitedly from foot to foot.

'Tell us, mummy, tells us please,' they chorused. 'Is he really not the puppy man, or is he just pretending?'

Steph took a long hard look at me, the bag, and then her two daughters. 'Yes girls,' she said at last, a slow smile spreading across her face as she took the bag from me. 'He was just pretending. He is the puppy man after all.'

I drove slowly home, stopping – in that politically incorrect fashion that members of my profession should never either adopt or encourage – for a cigarette at a vantage spot, looking back over Steph's valley. They didn't tell us about moments like this at medical school, but this is one I will still cherish until the end of my days.

Were I more in touch with my feminine side I would by now have had a lump in my throat and a warm glow somewhere to the left of my sternum. But it's just a job, I reminded myself. All in a day's work . . .

'Bloody hayfever,' I said out loud, dabbing my watering eyes with the back of my shirt sleeve.

11

We Thought it was All Over . . .

It was now two years after the opening of the new surgery, and by and large both the patients and I had adjusted to the changes I had instituted in the practice. Everything was running fairly smoothly – I had (mostly) adapted pretty well to an existence constantly under the spotlight, and the onerous demands of being forever on call.

But there remained one indisputable fly in the ointment . . .

I think it is fair to say, after due consideration of all the facts, in light of all the relevant circumstances, and after profound reflection upon the trials and tribulations of life as a rural GP, that an unassailable, pre-eminent truth had begun to emerge.

I absolutely hated taking Saturday morning surgery.

All right-minded people should spend their Saturday mornings leisurely recovering from the excesses of the Friday evening before. This is a delicate, time-consuming process requiring that absolute necessity for long life and happiness – a lie-in, or lay-in as it's known in these parts – followed by a preliminary amble through the Saturday papers, or at least, as many of the twenty-seven sections as you can get through in one sitting.

It's not surprising that we no longer have anaemic-looking, spindly-legged schoolboys doing the paper round but a combination of power lifters and marathon runners, each with their personal fitness trainer in tow. Most of our paper never makes it as far as the letter box these days, but is left like a sack of cement on the doorstep where we take it in turn to go and see if we can find the Sports section, before facing up to the daunting problem of recycling.

Pretty soon I think we shall just cut out the middle man, and have all our newspapers delivered straight to the paper-bank . . .

So, having lain in bed until the hangover finally shows early signs of abating, and waded through six hundred pages of travel, sport, weekend entertainment, appointments, personal finance and business – all the while wondering who has run off with the television pages – the search for the kettle begins. Once found, it's on to the coffee – and why *did* I leave it in the garden shed last night? – before moving on to the pivotal moment of the day. As the clock strikes twelve it is time for that most stalwart of party games, 'Hunt the Remote Control', hoping fervently you can find it before the start of *Football Focus*.

But Saturday morning surgery puts paid to all that.

While the rest of you are still emerging into the world wondering why you appear to be wearing somebody else's trousers, or hoping that you didn't really say what you think you might have done at the office party last night, we doctors are gingerly sitting down in our surgeries contemplating the usual unappetizing array of 'Emergencies Only' patients in the waiting room.

'Emergency', of course, is a quite specific piece of terminology meaning that something really important – in a medical sense only – is either going on right at this moment or will be happening within at least the next half-hour or so, before I depart on the visits. It will preferably be imminently life-threatening, involving quite a lot of severe pain and an acute shortness of breath, or at the very least entail the final stages of a long and exhausting labour culminating in the triumphant delivery of a set of triplets.

Consequently the waiting room should be a hive of noisy activity, with patients jostling competitively for positions at the front of the queue. The atmosphere will be redolent with un-pleasant smells, and you might confidently expect a good half of the occupants to be rolling around on our stain-resistant carpet howling in unbearable pain.

At least a quarter of those present should be bleeding profusely, a couple of them will be squabbling about who gets the vomit bowl first, and there should be at least one patient who does not move at all, their emergency having been so acute that they have actually died as a result of it whilst you were attending to the first of the three shotgun injuries laid out on makeshift stretchers in the surgery car park.

But somehow it is never quite like that.

You glance through the window into the waiting room and strangely, all is quiet. Mrs Barker is smiling quietly to herself as she reads 'Life's Like That' in the 1986 (June) edition of *Reader's Digest*, currently our most up-to-date volume, and Mr Armstrong-Jones is waiting patiently to have his ears syringed, having forgotten to attend his appointment with Katherine, the practice nurse, the day before. Ian Simpkins wants a sick note back-dated to a month last Thursday for an illness from which he has long since recovered and which neither I nor any other doctor actually witnessed, and the Robertson twins are playing in the toy pit — and, would you believe it, instead of crying uncontrollably and head-banging the skirting boards the little monsters are laughing and gurgling as contentedly as Winnie the Pooh might be whilst absconding with somebody else's full honey pot.

It is, in fact, business as usual. Armed with a mug of black coffee, a large wet flannel and a glass of water which has three of those round white things with some sort of paracetamol and codeine in, all of them fizzing far too noisily for my liking, I open the waiting-room door.

'Who's first?' I enquire incuriously.

They all look at me, and then look away again uneasily, each of them obviously reaching the no doubt sensible conclusion that one of their fellow sufferers should bear the initial brunt of my early morning testiness.

'OK,' I sigh wearily, 'no takers? Then what is it to be? Nearest the door? First person to wave a ten pound note in my direction? Anyone with intractable diarrhoea?

I am happy to report that this subtle, unchallenging approach to the proceedings often has the desired effect. The patients invariably shuffle uneasily in their seats until one of them submits to their inevitable fate, edging reluctantly towards my consulting room, a look of fear and trepidation on their face. Here, under cover of darkness and irrespective of the presenting complaint, I can wreak my revenge upon them. I find undertaking some totally unnecessary minor surgical procedure is always good for the soul, especially if it should involve a maximum of pain and suffering co-existent with a minimum of clinical benefit.

And if all else fails – step on their bunion. The resulting cries of agony, as they limp haltingly out of the door, should be enough to clear the waiting room for some time to come. But don't be misled . . . They will be back again, soon enough – hopefully *next* Saturday, with any luck, when my beleaguered partner, Dr Harper has the privilege of presiding over proceedings, but more probably in a fortnight, when I start all over again . . .

There are two other well-established ways of clearing a waiting room full of patients – and I should know, I've written a whole thesis upon it. Neither, I have to warn you, can be used on a regular basis.

Sooner or later, if you keep them waiting long enough, some elderly patient is bound to fall asleep. Do make sure that you pick one who isn't actually snoring.

Having carefully identified your victim look idly through the waiting-room window at them a couple of times, at first with a veneer of benevolent amusement on your face, following which you substitute a look of mild but growing concern. Next, send your receptionist out to bend attentively over the quietly reposing body, step back apace, gasping slightly, and then rush back to where you are trying unsuccessfully to compose yourself whilst hiding round the corner.

'Dr Sparrow,' she must say, just loudly enough to carry to the now increasingly apprehensive waiting room, 'it's poor Mrs Eastwick . . .'

You need do no more. They will all quietly slip away, tugging at their hankies and saying such things as 'And she made such a good Eccles cake, bless her,' 'What's going to happen to her parrot?' or 'But she looked so peaceful there, it was just as if she was asleep . . .'

OK, so it is going to be a teeny bit difficult explaining to the local practice population come Monday morning why Mrs Eastwick's parrot is still happily residing with the previously reported late Mrs Eastwick, but let's face it: if you've made it back home for *Football Focus* for the first time in six months, quite frankly . . . it's worth it.

The alternative scenario works only in a particular combination of circumstances.

First – and this is the easy bit – you need a hangover of monumental proportions, with all the trimmings. This should of necessity entail a complete set of red bleary eyes with bilaterally fixed pinhole pupils, a tongue stuck irrevocably to the roof of your mouth, and a slightly staggering gait, preferably with uncontrollable nausea.

Second, you need to be a doctor in Her Majesty's Armed Forces. Third – and most crucially – you need a waiting room full of young, impressionable cadets, with no one of any rank higher than yourself within possible earshot.

When all the relevant criteria are in place you then take centre stage, walking menacingly into the waiting room and standing as still as you are able – which probably isn't that still at all, but you trust they are too terrified to notice – until silence falls. Next you glare ferociously along the line of neatly scrubbed new recruits shuffling nervously on their seats in front of you, then sadistically sweep back along the line, frowning heavily, in the opposite direction.

Only when the last of them has stopped fidgeting do you begin to speak.

'I . . . ' you announce firmly, 'am your doctor. Yes, really,' fixing the eye of the most junior cadet whose look of surprise at your unexpected revelation is rather endearingly genuine, 'and I have to tell you that on this particular morning, when we are gathered here so joyously together, I feel unaccountably like some sort of precursor to death. Should any of you, when you finally get to enter my sympathetically low-level lighting consulting room, be deemed by what remains of my intellectual capabilities to be marginally less ill than myself, then you will automatically be on the most serious charge I can think of at the time. I don't as yet know which one that is likely to be, but I feel I should warn you that I have an exceptionally fertile imagination and a completely irrational approach to internal discipline.'

You then make to stagger tragically away but catch yourself in a moment of reconsideration, turning back once more with an afterthought. 'So I will be more than happy if all the really sick and needy amongst you stay – we can compare symptoms. The rest of you . . . '

It is, of course, a one-off situation.

RAF St Athan, South Wales, and it was spring, 1983.

Strange to say, within some thirty seconds of my adopting the above unconventional approach the entire waiting room had emptied. I stood, watching in relief through the waiting-room window as they dispersed to their respective parts of the station, only mildly perturbed by the poor unfortunate young man who seemed to be limping heavily into the distance on crutches I had a vague feeling he had not been in need of the previous morning.

One of the young medical administrative staff slipped unobtrusively up to my side, placing a vat of black coffee on the table.

He stood for a moment, watching through the window with me.

'Only a fractured fibula, sir,' he said, nodding in the direction of the crutches. 'Slipped over on the way to breakfast this morning, or so we are led to believe. Fortunately we had a spare pair of crutches in the office – Group Captain Marchmont's gout is subsiding again. Oh, and don't worry about the one on the far right of the group you can see, there, that chap being sick on the flower bed. An early appendicitis, sir, if you would like my opinion, but I'm sure he will keep until sir is suitably rehydrated. I took the liberty of making him another appointment to see you just after lunch.'

'Thank you, Simon,' I said humbly. 'Is there anything else I should be worrying about?'

'Well, there is the state of your shoes, sir. Would you like me to polish them now, or prepare the sugar and salt drip whilst you have a little lie-down in a darkened room?'

'What do you think, Simon?' I asked, crawling down the corridor towards the womb-like embrace of the ward.

'I'll go and get it set up for you now, sir,' he said calmly. 'That way it will be ready should we spot you lapsing into unconsciousness at an unanticipated moment. Keith has thoughtfully brought in his grandmother's commode . . . '

'Is his grandmother still on it?' I wondered.

'Not I think now, sir,' responded Simon, 'though Keith tells me that after rigor mortis had set in she is the only person he has ever heard of being buried in a sitting position. And we have all of us had a go with the bleach, sir, even Elaine and the cleaners . . . '

There is another, more soul-destroying part of the Saturday morning ritual in Lifton which takes place at precisely 11.45 a.m. The timing is crucial.

Any earlier and you can deal with it in plenty of time to return home at more or less the same time as your family are expecting you. Any later and your receptionist – if suitably bribed – can be coerced into pretending you have already left on an urgent visit.

'He won't be back before surgery closes down,' they are well primed to explain. 'Could you call back just after twelve o'clock when the deputizing service will have taken over? They'll be only too happy to help. I'm sure it could wait until then.'

Yes, you've guessed it.

11.45 a.m. on a Saturday morning is 'Request for a Totally Unnecessary Visit' time.

You just *know* that it is going to be a complete waste of your time, much as you just *know* you are going to have to undertake it anyway. So you grumble as much to your receptionist before reluctantly driving off to some obscure address out in the back of beyond and losing your way in a mobile phone dead zone. When you finally arrive at your intended destination, half an hour late and sweating and cursing profusely, the patient has either recovered and gone shopping or smiles sweetly at you from in front of the video and says, 'So nice of you to come, doctor, but it could have waited until Monday . . .'

How can you possibly respond without inviting litigation in a big way? How should you react when the suspected strangulated hernia turns out to be a truss put inadvertently on back to front?

'No problem, Mr Henderson. I was passing this way anyway.'

Pathetic, isn't it, how we all yearn so much to be loved that we meekly submit to the indignities of life that are continuously thrown at us?

It's Saturday morning in late August, and here is a typical example. My phone buzzed and I picked it up with my now almost permanent air of resignation.

'It's your 11.45 call,' said Sally, my receptionist, no doubt swiftly removing the receiver from her ear to ward off the worst of my subsequent violent explosion. I took the call with the complete lack of interest that even a couple of years in general practice imbues upon you, if you survive it that long.

'I want you to come and see my father,' came the clipped, well-modulated tones of a middle-aged man with just a hint of superiority in his voice. It was that 'I'm a very important cog in middle management whilst you are simply a rural GP' inflection that I find so appallingly irritating. But I hid it well, I like to think.

'Why?' I asked politely. 'Is he particularly aesthetically pleasing upon the eye? Does he have a once in a lifetime rash, a never to be seen again discharge, a catch it whilst you can suppurating ulcer? Is he –'

'You obviously failed to qualify at the school of charm,' responded the well-modulated tones icily, 'but if you are all that there is, then you will just have to do. My father has acute chest pain, which is now going down his left arm. I may not be a doctor but I know enough to realize it sounds like a heart attack. I want you to come and see him this instant.'

I so nearly said, 'Could it not wait until after *Football Focus*?' but decided that even for me there are times when discretion should take precedence over abject stupidity. This may possibly have had something to do with the fact that people with chest pain going down their left arm just occasionally really are having a heart attack, and some people having heart attacks have been known to die.

And if that wasn't enough to stir me into action, a recently published general practice survey had found that all people with clipped, well-modulated tones whose fathers die of a heart attack whilst the GP is watching the television in preference to visiting can be guaranteed to sue, and will invariably succeed.

'I'm on my way,' I said briskly, reassuring myself that if I drove really fast I might just get back in time for Goal of the

Season, and ran out to the office where Sally was waiting soberly, holding a set of notes in her hand.

'I knew you would be going,' she said. 'He spoke awfully well, didn't he?'

'Awfully,' I agreed, and walked past her before stopping to say, 'Am I really that predictable?'

'Oh, it's not that,' she said, smiling sweetly. 'But he is the sort that would sue, isn't he?'

I collected my drug bag, some needles, a syringe or two, a stethoscope and that thing you look up people's noses with — you never know when it might come in handy. Bundling them carelessly into the cardboard box I generally use for my rounds — which I subsequently hid judiciously in the boot (first impressions count, you know) — I drove off rapidly into the midday sun.

Although I had not previously met my patient-to-be — Dr Harper had always dealt with him before — I knew more or less where he lived. Twenty minutes later I pulled up in the drive of the house, breathing heavily, having rapidly traversed the barren northern wastelands of the practice, and knocked on the front door. Nobody answered. I knocked on the back door, and again nobody answered.

I knocked on the side door, the kitchen window, opened the conservatory, looked through the lounge doors and walked down to the garden shed. I walked round the back of the house, the side, the front again and the other side, even going down to the greenhouse, which was pretty pointless really as I could see all the way through it from the top of the lawn and knew perfectly well it was empty. Still nobody answered, and all chance of making *Football Focus* was fading into oblivion.

I walked round the house one last time, found a ladder and scaled it to look through a second-floor window, shinned down a drainpipe, swung from the chandeliers, swam a couple of lengths in the swimming pool and played happily for half an hour on the croquet lawn. Still nobody came.

In final, sheer frustration I battered and battered on the front door, and then sank to my knees on the doorstep, raising my arms helplessly to the heavens. I had had enough.

'You stupid, stupid, *stupid* man,' I shouted in utter frustration. 'What's the point of calling me out here for some potentially life-threatening condition and then not being in to be bloody well life-threatened by it?'

There was a discreet cough behind me, and I spun around in surprise. A middle-aged, smooth-looking chap in an expensive suit that I just knew had to be Mr Clipped and Well-Modulated Tones had climbed out of his car (that is his big, expensive and very, *very* quiet car) and stood looking down his no doubt expensively reupholstered nose, saying haughtily:

'Actually, he is in. He's just not in here. That . . . ' and he jabbed his forefinger in the direction of the only other house anywhere within sight, 'is where he is in, and where you currently are not. I just hope for your sake he's not dying.'

'You and me both,' I muttered viciously. 'You and me both.'

Father of Mr Clipped and Well-Modulated Tones – now rapidly transforming into Mr Clipped, Very Angry and Increasingly Litigatious by the Moment – did at first sight look rather ill, I have to say. Fortunately for me I was the only doctor present, with no one to contradict me. *Football Focus* was sadly long since over, and there was no further need for any haste. I reached for my stethoscope, wondering if I could put the thing for looking up people's noses to a more enterprising use.

Very Angry met me as I descended the stairs after finishing my examination. 'Well, doctor, have you formed an opinion?' he asked officiously. 'Do you know what you are going to do, how to respond, where we are going from here? Will you be summoning an ambulance?' he asked, adding darkly, 'If it is not already too late for us all, by now.'

I furrowed my brow in mock concentration before giving my considered assessment.

'Yes, I have,' I said slowly. 'You, sir, are a pillock, I'm going home, and you should go and get hold of a kite.'

'A kite?' he said, visibly taken aback.

One of the reasons I have done so well – and survived so long – in general practice is my unfailing ability to respond with tact and diplomacy in the most delicate of situations.

'Yes, a kite,' I reiterated, 'because you and your father both have more than enough wind to go fly it.'

Saturday morning again, two weeks later. It was now 11.40, and all was going well.

It had been a quiet surgery, although no one had dared say so. Quiet is a word which is strictly banned in our building.

'Isn't it quiet?' some unguarded soul will say, and you can bet a lifetime supply of white chocolate Magnums that within a matter of minutes a coachload of senior citizens on the last day of their mystery tour from Clacton-on-Sea will turn up in the surgery car park with acute gastro-enteritis, before emerging vomiting and haemorrhaging internally all over our front lawn.

But it had – dare I say it – been peaceful, a chance for once to get in an hour's paperwork before heading for home. I had promised the kids they could go on a bike ride that afternoon – nothing unusual in that, you might think, but this time I had promised I would even go with them. A simple enough aspiration for most people, but one which meant getting home on time, which meant leaving the surgery on time, which meant, please God, for once, forgoing the ritualistic torture of the 11.45 phone call.

An hour's paperwork, I should here explain, means ten minutes deciding which of the really big piles to consign unread to the shredder, forty-five minutes attending to the evil deed, two minutes opening the post and the remaining three minutes answering the inevitable questionnaires that bombard us poor overworked, under-appreciated, over-stressed and under-re-munerated general practitioners.

And if you think my description appears a touch self-pitying, then you are of course totally correct, but just how would *you* respond to 125-page questionnaire entitled 'How to Reduce the Volume of Paperwork in General Practice?'

We are often asked to report back various meaningless statistics to the health authority – the number of complaints we have received in a year, for example, and more recently the number of plaudits.

'I think I once had a "God, you were wonderful, "' said Dr Harper, after considering thoughtfully, 'but I'm not all that sure it was from a patient.'

I have now resolved the paperwork problem once and for all. When the pile on my desk in front of me became so high I could no longer see the patients over it I embarked on a revolutionary crusade. We took all the surgery furniture to the local authority dump and fashioned some papier-mâché desks, chairs and a rather attractive chaise-longue out of the vast natural resources available to us . . .

In my former RAF days, a Squadron Leader pilot of my acquaintance had an innovative approach to the paperwork he felt under-stimulated to deal with. After a few moments' perusal he merely stamped it 'Official Bullshit' in bright red ink and instructed his secretary to return it immediately to whence it came.

The Air Force, being relentlessly unforgiving, duly assigned him to the worst fate known to man – three years in charge of a dozen other men of like-minded mentality and a complete inability to fly a fast jet in the same direction for more than a few seconds at any one time.

They had a collective name for this group of misfits that I can only vaguely remember. I can still see them in their funny crimson-red boiler suits, blond highlights in their hair and designer shades before they became fashionable – what was it again?

Ah yes – the Red Arrows, that was it.

Questionnaires are of course supremely relevant to general practice, and without question help us in our eternal quest to consistently improve our clinical techniques. We greet their arrival with unfailing enthusiasm, and if more than two of us are present, an ecstatic round of applause.

'How many of your patients have wigs that are truly in keeping with their ethnic origins?' asked one, kindly sent to us by a research analyst from Southampton. For some reason I have never been able to fully explain why all such mindlessly banal publications seem to emanate from the south coast. Why should this be?

I blame career advisers myself. 'Got a degree in analytical research from Grantham Polytechnic?' I can hear them saying. 'Then Bournemouth is the place for you.' It is no doubt part of some sinister government plot to bore the local geriatric population to the earliest possible demise and reduce the community nursing and social security budget, because, as we all know, the cheapest patient to run is a dead one. And it works, apparently.

Well, I ask you, how on earth am I supposed to know what ghastly National Health wigs my patients have had inflicted upon them? I might just spot an Afro-Caribbean inappropriately attired in some carrot-topped paraphernalia, but ninety-three-year-old ladies with thinning grey hair that looks as if it has been put on backwards in a thunderstorm are two a penny in our practice. And what about extravagantly hirsute babies that have been fitted with bald skull caps to enable them to merge more unobtrusively with their follicularly challenged peer groups? How am I supposed to know?

In all honesty, I am only fully aware of one of my patients who wears a wig, and that is indisputably Mr Parkinson. You need not be academically gifted to spot it – an eighty-five-year-old man with a sparse grey rim of wispy nothingness crowned by a ginger nylon creation from the Ambrosia lost property department just stands up and begs to be noticed. The only good thing I can say about it is that nobody in our village has the least idea whether he has put it on the right way round or not.

Mr Parkinson, now sadly deceased, lived but a few hundred yards from the surgery – a few hundred yards, and a few hundred hours to travel the distance between the two. Watching him struggle down to our door was akin to watching grass grow in the depths of winter, but without quite so much of the action.

He was the proud owner of what can be loosely described as a dog – at least, I think it started life out as a dog but it had since mutated into a small asthmatic rug on legs with a pronounced inability to recall in which direction it was supposed to be walking.

It had to happen. One windy morning, Mr Parkinson and dog were shuffling painfully down the road towards the surgery, though this being pension day they had probably initially set out for the post office but had taken a left at the front door instead of a right, and it was just too much effort to turn round. This would not be the first such occasion this had happened, and for his benefit alone we had reached a mutually acceptable agreement with the village postmistress. We would sell the occasional stamp and some middle of the range stationery, and they had a complete array of our most popular suppositories. Everybody was happy, especially Mr Parkinson, who could then purchase his two most important everyday commodities at either end of the village without worrying.

So the wind blew, and the Sellotape, Airfix glue or reconstituted chewing gum that was used to attach hairpiece to head proved sadly unequal to the task. Mr Parkinson and his wig parted company, to the never to be forgotten delight of the junior school immediately adjacent to our surgery whose aspiring criminal fraternity were loitering by the gate with intent, although at this tender age they would not yet be sure what intent it was they were loitering with.

'Fetch, Rex,' bellowed Mr Parkinson in a hitherto completely unanticipated roar.

Where did he get the lungs for it? I wondered idly, for a second scouring the street for the accompanying portable ventilation machine. And then for one insane, surreal moment, I visualized that the wig might come scurrying back, collect Rex by the scruff of the neck and drop him eagerly in our waiting room, panting with thoroughly deserved pride in a difficult and wholly unexpected deed most efficiently executed.

But no. More incredible even than that, Rex turned tail and hared down the road in the wake of the rapidly departing hairpiece, his little legs a blur of action. It was more beautiful a moment than *One Man and his Dog* has ever encapsulated, especially given their advantage of having the grudging assistance of a few tatty sheep and a couple of five-barred gates.

I witnessed all this from my waiting-room window, and being above all a man with a mission to tend the sick and the needy I went out into the road to offer what assistance I could. Not to mention to get a better view.

It was dustbin day, and let us be charitable, Rex was probably confused. Call it his cataracts, his increasing lack of smell, or the natural befuddlement of his inexorably advancing years, but when he came back, tail wagging feverishly and a grin of joyous companionship you could never forget etched from ear to whiskery ear, he deposited at his master's feet not an appallingly prescribed nylon wig, but a scrap of what I suspect once used to be an orangey-brown carpet I had previously noticed languishing outside number 22 Orchard Close in the hope that one of the refuse executives (yes, I do mean the dustmen) might be charitable for once and chuck it in the back of the van.

There have been many times in my career when I have truly not known how to react, and every now and then one of these occurs when I do not unfortunately have a drink in my hand to resort to. This was one such of those.

I looked down at Rex, and then across to Mr Parkinson, and for a fleetingly awful moment I thought that I wanted to laugh. But I am still occasionally humbled by the unexpected dignity of one of my patients, and never more so than now.

'Well, Rex,' said Mr Parkinson in a purely man-to-dog interchange, 'how lucky I am to have you to look after me.' And with that he bent down arthritically, grasped the decaying piece of carpet as if it were two new hips and a pacemaker and planted it firmly upon his head. Rex was positively glowing with pride.

'Oh, I may be old,' said Mr Parkinson, looking directly across at me, 'but I'm not stupid. I know they all laugh at me,' nodding in the direction of the school, 'and nice doctor though I know that you are, I expect you laugh at me a little too, once in a while . . . '

I just hoped his rheumy eyes failed to spot me blushing to the roots of my hair.

' . . . but I love my dog, and he loves me, and that is more important to us both than anything the rest of you might think of us.'

He turned and beckoned to his devoted friend. 'Come on, Rex,' he said gently, 'time to be getting along,' and they carried on walking slowly down the road, side by side.

I swear I heard echoing behind him, with a self-deprecating chuckle, 'We'll be down at your place, in a while. Stamps and suppositories, if you please, just as usual . . . '

It's 11.41, and blessed silence still reigns.

'The telephone's been disconnected,' I fantasized out loud. 'An earthquake has struck this side of Exeter and everyone is evacuating before the tidal wave comes. A black hole has materialized over Bristol . . . '

'Maybe it's just no one is ill,' rejoined Sally. 'I do realize it's a Saturday morning but it can happen, you know.'

'Don't be stupid,' I expostulated. 'Come back to earth and be more realistic – for every person who really is ill, there are at least a couple of dozen who simply think they are, and most of them live in Lewdown . . . '

11.42, and I'm holding my breath.

Still holding, but now I'm going a bit blue round the edges.

11.44, and the phone rings. 'Ha,' ejaculated Sally, 'two minutes early. Haven't started on my cream bun, yet.'

11.45, and she puts the phone down. 'Wrong number,' she explains, 'following up one of your failures. They wanted the undertakers.'

11.46 . . . 11.47 . . . Silence continues blissfully to reign.

11.48 sails past wholly uninterrupted, and as the last second of 11.49 ticks by it finds me whistling happily in the dispensary.

At the end of 11.50, the whistling suddenly stops.

'It's the Countryman's Arms,' mumbled Sally indistinctly through her second cream bun. 'They want you to go and see someone there.'

'Tell them I'm having a nervous breakdown. Or the dog's died, or the surgery's on fire, or I'm needed urgently at the Millennium Dome. Tell them anything.'

Sally considered carefully for a moment. 'You had a nervous breakdown a fortnight ago, you don't currently have a dog, the surgery has been razed to the ground at least half a dozen times since I have been here, only to be miraculously restored by the following morning, and you don't even know where the Millennium Dome is.'

'Other receptionists lie for their doctors,' I said pitifully, 'at other surgeries.'

'But I don't work at any other surgery,' she answered sweetly, passing me the phone. 'I work at this one.'

I gave in. 'Yes, what do you want?' I asked good-naturedly. 'An emergency carbuncle, perhaps? Head cook lost a fingernail in the lasagne? Sudden outbreak of –'

'Shut up, Mike,' came the unflustered tones of Robert, the Countryman's owner. 'Look, I know you're probably just about

253

to go off duty, but could you come and take a look at one of our residents?'

'And why should I?' I demanded, not in the slightest bit reasonably. 'Has he got two heads or something? Green slime oozing from his nostrils? Recently ashore from the *Marie Celeste* and you want a quarantine certificate? Is he – '

'God, you do go on, don't you? Be serious, if you possibly can for a moment. I don't think he's very well.'

'And what does he think?'

'Mike, please don't mess around. Look, this chap called in yesterday afternoon, not from around here, said he didn't feel too good and went straight to bed. This morning he's rung through for three jugs of orange juice to be left outside his door, and I just went over to check on him but he's not answering. We've tried ringing the room, but he won't answer the phone either. His car's still here, though, parked outside the door. Mike, I'm worried – please come over and see what's going on.'

It was the 'Mike, I'm worried' bit that did it. They never rang without good reason – the last time being over two years previously when a middle-aged man had a choking fit in the dining room and all but died before he had even ordered dessert. It was all most unfortunate – quite put the rest of the diners off their meals, and he was rushed off to hospital without paying the bill.

I am a GP. I have a calling, a mission to heal, a duty to serve. I decided to go.

After all, there might be a free pint in it.

The small country hotel was only a couple of miles up the road from the surgery, and I pulled up into the courtyard just as the church clock struck eleven. It wasn't actually eleven o'clock, of course – this being a church in a tiny hamlet in the middle of nowhere – it was just striking eleven, and I would defend its right to do so to anyone.

I glanced at the clock in the car and groaned inwardly. I just hoped the kids would understand.

Robert came out to meet me, a jovial, ruddy-faced man with a cook's pot belly and a small goatee beard that should have looked ridiculous, but which he somehow managed to get away with. He rubbed his hands together as if warming some Blu-Tack prior to sticking up the Saturday evening menu.

'Thanks for coming, Mike. Kettle's on, when you've finished. He's over there,' pointing up the hill, 'chalet four. That's his car outside, the blue Peugeot.'

'Have you been in yourself?' I asked mildly. 'And did he ask for vodka and Galliano as well – he might have been making a lifetime's supply of Harvey Wallbangers, might he not?'

'Er, not actually in,' he admitted, shifting from foot to foot uneasily. 'Bit squeamish, you understand. I'm fine with an unplucked pheasant or a yet to be gutted salmon, but not all that hot with other people's illnesses. Pain, vomiting, that sort of thing.'

'Right,' I said with a mock sigh.

'But I have brought the keys for you,' he continued, beaming cherubically and dangling them enticingly before me, 'and I do have some bacon sizzling on the hot plate, a newly laid egg which is still warm on the outside, and a bottle of something fresh from the cellar, something dark, woody and expensive with the cork just begging to be pulled.'

'How woody?' I asked grudgingly.

'Seriously woody,' he said, his eyes sparkling, 'with a nose you can smell a mile the other side of a howling gale.'

'Just give me the room keys,' I said, 'and I'll be with you as soon as I can. By the way, what's his name?'

'He registered as a Mr Jeffries, but I'm not so sure it's his real name, for some reason. From up your way, somewhere in the Midlands – Kettering, that's it. Oh, and these are his car keys, if you need them. He left them at reception.'

'Thanks,' I said sardonically, slipping them into my pocket. 'I'm sure they'll come in really useful. Now go and see to the bacon, there's a good chap. Wouldn't want it to be burning without you.'

I walked up the short hill to the row of chalets nestling in the midday sun, my mind more on the bicycle and children I wasn't approaching than the patient I was. I knocked on the door, and when there was no answer, I knocked again.

'Mr Jeffries,' I called, 'I'm the . . .' My voice faded away, some instinct telling me there was to be no response forthcoming.

The key turned easily in the door, and I pushed it open to reveal a small but immaculately clean and tidy room that at first sight appeared empty, but at second was indisputably not. A radio played softly in the background, and lying motionless on the bed before me lay the inert body of a man in perhaps his early thirties. I held my breath and took a few tentative steps forward, relaxing perceptibly as I realized he was alive, although his breathing was shallow and laboured, his colour high, and the room had a slightly sweet smell.

Not a well man, I thought quickly. He had a fever, too, as I touched his forehead with the back of my hand and recoiled as if scalded. Hot, young, unconscious – the spectre of meningitis reared in my mind. Or malaria, maybe, or even rabies? I scanned his body quickly for rashes. Should I rush off and get myself immunized against something – or indeed everything – right this minute and come back only when suitably protected against anything contagious, with six layers of polythene and a riot shield?

I put a hand on his shoulder instead, and shook him gently. He might have just been asleep, but he wasn't, he was comatose, and I shook him and shook him some more until a look of irritation flitted across his unshaven features and he opened his eyes briefly.

'Mr Jeffries,' I said quietly, 'I'm Dr Sparrow. I'm one of the local GPs around here.'

He closed his eyes again, and just as I thought he was drifting back into unconsciousness he said, 'Don't need a doctor,' slurring his words slightly, 'Jus' need to sleep. I'm all right. No doctor, no medicines, I'm all right. Jus' leave me alone.'

'Can't do that, Mr Jeffries,' I said firmly. 'Look, I can't keep calling you Mr Jeffries. What's your first name?'

He was drifting again, and I reclaimed my hold on his shoulder, shaking him once more.

'Not Jeffries,' he said finally. 'Gave a false name. Don't come from Kettering, either. Don't want anyone to know where I am. Just want to sleep. Left alone and sleep.'

It was an effort for him to talk, but an effort I knew he had to keep making.

'What's your first name, then?' I asked. 'You can tell me that, can't you?'

His eyes, bloodshot and pitted, opened briefly

'Colin,' he said, wincing as a spasm of pain shot through him.

'Colin what?' I persisted.

'Just Colin,' he said. 'Just Colin, Just William, Just Colin, Just William. Just Colin,' and he laughed humourlessly.

'And your surname?'

'Just Colin,' he repeated. 'Don't want anyone to know where I am. Don't want any help. Just want to sleep, and to . . .'

He mumbled something indistinctly, and suddenly it hit me. This wasn't an illness, after all.

'Colin,' I said gently, 'have you taken something?'

Tears welled in his tightly shut eyes, and gradually I managed to piece the story together. His business had failed, his wife had left with the children, and twenty-four hours earlier he had taken over a hundred paracetamol, travelling far enough away from home to be unrecognized, and with only one intent in mind.

He had come here to die, and I feared he was going to succeed.

'I have to get you into hospital,' I said. 'And soon.'

'No, no hospital,' he pleaded feebly, 'don't want to go to

hospital. Don't want anyone to know. Can't you just leave me here, leave me alone . . ?'

When all else fails there remains one tool of the trade to which you can always turn, a tool of the below belt, knife in the back variety.

Emotional blackmail, and this seemed to be the time to use it.

'Have you got children, Colin?' I asked.

He nodded, barely perceptibly.

'What must they be feeling?' I continued, 'worrying about where you are? They'll need their father, Colin, whatever you think now they will need you to be there, one day. I can't just walk away and leave you, whatever you may want. I have to act for your children, Colin, because there is nobody else here to do it for them at the moment.'

And of course, although I did not actually say it, GPs who leave an obviously dying man to go on a bike ride with their offspring just because the dying man asked them to do so tend to have fairly poor career prospects, in the long term.

Colin didn't argue any more, because he had lapsed back into unconsciousness. I left the chalet, ran back down to the main building, and asked for the phone.

'Problems?' asked Robert quietly, taking one look at my face and reading it correctly.

'Yeah,' I nodded. 'Big ones. One very unwell patient, and two soon to be very disappointed children.' But at least my kids would be there tomorrow, I thought, though as for Colin . . .

I rang for an ambulance, and I rang home to explain, and then I sat out in the sunshine to wait, chewing reflectively on a bacon sandwich, reflecting on how harsh and unforgiving life could sometimes be.

Twenty minutes later I heard the siren echoing down the valley, and shortly afterwards came the reassuring sight of the ambulance as it rounded the corner and hove into view, screeching to a halt in the courtyard. A couple of windows in the hotel opened as the residents began to appreciate there was a drama being played out before their eyes. This was much more exciting than watching the cows being milked.

The crew disembarked, one, Barry, that I knew well from frequent encounters over the years, the other a young woman I had not seen before.

'Hiyah, Mike,' called Barry, comfortingly professional as he busied himself in the back of the ambulance. 'This is Alexandra, known as Alex, up from Truro for the day to see how we manage things in the real world.'

'In other words to give them a hand,' smiled Alex, 'and bring a little culture and sophistication into their otherwise drab and meaningless lives.'

'Where's our patient?' asked Barry, emerging with a profusion of oxygen cylinders, tangled tubing and orange bags full of equipment I could not even pronounce, let alone endeavour to use with anything approaching competence.

'In there,' I nodded, 'but he doesn't want to play. I haven't actually figured out how we're going to get him into the ambulance, as yet, because he doesn't want to go. He doesn't even know you're here, in fact. And he's comfortable, he wants to die, and he seems to have found the right place to do it.'

'Aggressive?'

'Not yet, but I guess he could be. And people always look so much smaller when they're lying down, don't they?'

We walked into chalet four, Barry, Alex and I, to see what we were going to do, and in an instant what we were going to do changed irrevocably.

'Oh my God,' said Alex faintly, on seeing the inert body lying before us, 'it's Colin Bowyer. Can we go and talk outside for a moment?'

'I was at school with him,' she said, as we emerged blinking into the sunlight. 'You never think that people you were at school with will make the news, do you, but he's been on all the local radio and TV programmes for the past twenty-four hours.'

Light was beginning to dawn on Barry, though not on me. 'You mean that's . . ?' he said in wonderment.

'He's wanted in connection with abducting a twelve-year-old child,' said Alex. 'I'm not sure who, they didn't say, but they've been broadcasting details of him, and his car . . . '

'That's the one you're leaning on now, Mike,' put in Barry helpfully.

' . . . and saying if you see either of them to contact the police immediately,' continued Alex. 'Fancy that, Colin Bowyer, after all these years . . . '

It all became rather frenetic, after that. Barry radioed for the police, Robert shepherded his guests out of the hotel and away from the action, I rang home and said I was going to be even later than anticipated, and then Robert brought out tea, and biscuits, and some rather nice cake.

I am constantly struck by how the bizarre slips so easily into the commonplace, in general practice, and the commonplace into the bizarre. If you could have seen us there, taking tea and biscuits in the midday sun, in the sleepiest of Devon hamlets while the county's most wanted man lay semi-comatose just a few yards away, you would begin to understand.

So we sat, and we supped, and we waited in the still country air, until suddenly all hell was let loose. A fleet of police cars, a couple more ambulances, two helicopters circling overhead, noise, confusion, dust, and heat, and everywhere uniformed officers, with more mobile phones than you would see at a telecommunications convention.

And then, just as suddenly, they were all gone, and the still and the quiet began to settle on our valley once more. As the last vehicle pulled away, as the last uniform disappeared out of sight, Robert puffed his way up the hill to where I rested contemplatively on the bonnet of the notorious blue Peugeot.

'You're a wonderful man, Robert Urquhart,' I said with feeling, as he passed me a glass of the red woody stuff he had promised seemingly light years ago, 'and thank goodness that's all over.'

He perched on the bonnet beside me. 'Well, all publicity is good for business,' he said easily. 'What had he actually done, that chap?'

And then, as I realized where we were, and what he had done, and on what we were sitting, I could feel the colour suddenly drain from my face. I put my hand in my pocket and drew out a set of car keys that did not belong to me.

'Oh my God,' said Robert quietly. 'It's not all over, is it?

We both arose, walked to the rear of the car, and stood looking, and hoping, and trying not to think. I took two steps forward, and put the key in the lock.

And then I opened the boot.

But the boot was empty.

Truth, as it is said, is so often stranger than fiction.

I heard from Robert, several months later, that Colin had been transferred to a hospital in the North, where he had undergone a liver transplant. I heard, too, that subsequently he had died.

And of the girl? I never found out.

On the Saturday in question the West Country police were looking for two men, one who had kidnapped a twelve-year-old girl, and the other, a lonely, depressed family man whose wife desperately wanted his safe return. Somehow, in the confusion that had arisen between the broadcasters and police the two wanted men had merged into one.

And our man, Colin, had simply come here to die.

12

Exercising My . . .

'One thing you must never do,' an eminent professor told us early in our student careers, fresh-faced and innocent as we were, 'is lie to your patients.'

Yes, you – like me – have a feeling we've been here before.

The words 'Why not?' sprang immediately to mind, but that was not what actually came next.

'May we then be economical with the truth, sir?' asked Declan politely in his lazy Irish drawl, obviously a politician in the making.

'You, O'Shaughnessy,' countered the professor, peering not unkindly over his half-moon spectacles, 'will no doubt elevate it into an art form, given any available opportunity, but in answer to your question, no. You should be neither economical with the truth nor even just a touch parsimonious.'

'And why is that, sir?' asked Declan, apparently in self-destruct mode. 'Just so that I shall know for future reference, you understand.'

'Firstly,' responded the professor firmly, 'because it is both ethically and professionally unsound. Secondly – and more importantly – sooner or later your patients will find you out, and slowly but surely their faith in you will be gradually undermined. And when that begins to happen, young man, then you are finished, and finished for good.'

He paused for a moment, and sat on the edge of his desk at the front of the lecture theatre as the weight of his words sank in.

'Lies are like a cancer,' he continued. 'They may rest undetected for a while, but eventually they will grow, spreading stealthily throughout your body until they erupt like a secondary deposit in the spinal cord, just when you are least expecting it.'

We all sat, and pondered upon his words. All, that is, except one of us.

'Then why sir,' persisted Declan, completely unabashed, 'did you tell that old lady on Michigan Ward last Tuesday that you had managed to remove every last vestige of her bowel tumour when you operated on her the day before?'

The lecture theatre became suddenly quiet, as the professor considered his response with the same sort of concentration as Declan now began to consider his future. The professor, normally a man of benign temperament, was renowned for his occasional unpredictable explosions and intermittent vitriolic pursuits of students he took a particular dislike to.

A collective stillness hung over the lecture room. Even Declan, insouciant chap that he was, began to look pale. In his defence, I have to say that I don't believe his question was meant to be anything other than innocuous. Misguided and full of abject stupidity, I grant you, but innocuously misguided and stupidly abject. Everyone held their breath. Well, almost everyone.

There's always one, isn't there?

'Is that what you call "exercising your clinical judgement"?' I asked innocently.

So, should we actually tell the truth, the whole truth and nothing but the truth on each and every occasion?

'Tell me doctor, honestly,' a patient might say. 'Am I going to die soon?'

It is a far from unusual question, and there are a range of responses one can produce.

Option 1: To be used sparingly – in other words only when there is insufficient time for the patient to ring his lawyer, a close friend or a relative. Look at him thoughtfully, glance casually down at your watch and say, 'So what do you mean by soon?'

Option 2: Which is just a little more callous, is to say 'Yup,' and move on quickly to the next patient.

Option 3: The more subtle approach. 'Have you ever read *War and Peace?*' I might enquire occasionally, to be followed – according to the response – by 'Good, then that's one thing you won't be missing out on,' or, with a sad shake of the head, 'Well, I'm afraid it's too late for that now.'

Or you can just lie blatantly, in as reassuring a manner as possible, along the lines of: 'Don't worry, Mr Arnold. We're doing everything we can. Just relax now, and everything will be fine.'

So is lying to our patients ever permissible? And if so, in what circumstances, and who makes the decision?

I leave you to judge . . .

Mary Smith was in her late sixties, and had bowel cancer. I knew, her daughter knew, even her two-year-old granddaughter and half the village knew, and I think most of their herd of prize Friesians had a pretty good idea of it, too.

Mary, however, did not have a clue.

She had had what used to be called a nervous breakdown in her mid-forties, spending several months as a voluntary admission in the local psychiatric home, which has now been razed to the ground and is currently reincarnated as the organic section of the frozen food department in the local Tesco's. Mary unfortunately lived on the knife edge of an acute anxiety that could topple into a deep depression with just the minimum of prompting.

I rather think the words 'I have to tell you that you're dying, Mary,' might have done it.

She had lost weight recently and was passing blood in her stools. Her daughter brought her in to see me.

'I do hope it's nothing too serious, doctor,' Mary said nervously, twisting her handkerchief round and round in her hands.

'I'm sure it won't be,' I replied, as reassuringly as possible. 'I just need to run a few tests on you, Mary, that's all.'

I sat reviewing the results several days later, and my heart sank. Mary was profoundly anaemic, and the probable diagnosis was disturbing. I referred her urgently to one of the local surgeons, a friend of mine for many years.

'I'm sure it's nothing to worry about, Mary,' I reassured her again when she next visited. 'Just a few more tests to run. They probably seem interminable to you, but we just want to do everything properly, that's all.'

'Whatever you say, doctor,' she said, grasping my hand. 'You know how much I trust you. Whatever you say is fine by me.'

A barium enema and a colonoscopy later, the stark evidence was staring us in the face. They had found a lesion in her bowel which needed urgent removal.

'For God's sake don't mention the word "cancer",' I begged the surgeon before he saw her again. 'Don't even let it pass through your mind whilst she's still in the room. She's almost psychic – one hint of the dreaded diagnosis and we'll be scraping her off the sidewalk within a fortnight. And avoid the word "biopsy", if you can – just use "polyp" followed by the phrase "and we'll get rid of it for you", in your most reassuring fashion. Please?'

He was a sensible man, the surgeon – or still in need of my private referrals – because he did precisely as I asked. When the result of Mary's histology came back he made sure it was sent to me to pass on the news as I saw fit, instead of poor Mary waiting in fear and trepidation for her next outpatient appointment, as would have otherwise been the case.

She came into my surgery the next week with her daughter, as usual, looking pale and worried.

'What news have you got for me, doctor?' she asked nervously, a tremor in her right hand. 'Is everything going to be all right?'

I looked at the histology report on the piece of paper in front of me. 'Poorly differentiated adenocarcinoma of the colon,' I read, 'with diffuse early local spread.'

In other words, cancer of the bowel and about as nasty as it could get, although still in a reasonably early stage.

'Never lie to your patients,' rang the professor's words in my head. 'Lies are like a tumour . . . sooner or later you will be found out . . . '

'Everything's fine, Mary,' I lied unblinkingly. 'Just a boring old polyp. You'll live to be a hundred.'

'You mean there isn't any . . . I haven't got . . . ' Mary's voice faltered.

'None at all,' I continued shamelessly.

Her eyes lit up, and a little colour came back to her cheeks.

'Oh,' she said, 'I'm so pleased. I can stop worrying now. Thank you so much, doctor, I'm so lucky to have you to look after me, aren't I, Bessie?' turning to her daughter. 'Someone I can trust.'

Over the next few years Mary would come to see me intermittently, always seeming to be miraculously free from any further problems.

If she mentioned it at all she would refer to her spell under the surgeons as 'my little bit of trouble', leaving the consulting room with something along the lines of 'So lucky to have you, doctor,' or 'Having someone I can trust is so important, don't you think?'

Each time she had an appointment at the outpatient department in our local hospital to see the surgeon, Bessie would ring me a few days in advance.

'She's off up to Launceston again next week,' she would say. 'Please could you ring them, just to be sure?' and I would phone through to explain.

'Please don't tell Mary Smith she has cancer, no matter what she might ask you,' I would plead, and each time the new senior house officer, or registrar — and sometimes even the consultant himself, putting in an unexpected appearance — would agree without question.

I suppose it had to happen, sooner or later.

Some five years after her initial diagnosis I received a phone call from Mary's daughter.

'She's not well, Dr Sparrow, I'm afraid. I'm no expert but I think she's looking a bit jaundiced, and she's lost an awful lot of weight in the last few weeks. I know it had to happen one day, but . . . poor Mum. I don't want her to suffer.'

'Has she said anything?' I asked, knowing the answer before I spoke.

'Not a word. Just that she felt a bit tired this morning and thought she might stay in bed for a while.'

I promised to visit after branch surgery, and rang off.

Branch surgery (the one in the lavatory) was a simple enough affair as my only patients were two children with runny noses and a repeat prescription of her heart failure drugs for Emma — not exactly a patient as such, but old Mrs Bulstrode's much-loved border terrier. Mrs Bulstrode, as I was well aware, could no longer afford the vet's fees, and what the NHS doesn't know . . .

Work over, I drove thoughtfully back into town . . . shortly afterwards driving thoughtfully back again, having forgotten to visit Mary as intended.

This absent-mindedness of mine is becoming sadly more common than it used to be. In my early years as a GP I would never forget a visit, a name or where to insert a suppository, but nowadays if I remember both my own name and which day of the week it is at one and the same time I feel strangely cheered.

Only the other day — and I swear this is true — I left a patient in my consulting room for a moment while I nipped out to my car to get my stethoscope, which was still in there from my late night visit the previous evening.

On the way back I was waylaid in reception for a minute, answered a phone call, gave some unsolicited advice over the counter on how to deal with persistent thread-worms, glanced quickly in the visit book and shot out to see an elderly woman living in the furthest reaches of the practice who was suffering from the first of her two-monthly winter bronchitis attacks. Three-quarters of the way there I remembered the patient in my consulting room, still waiting . . .

This may, of course, be merely a country phenomenon. Our local vicar, Paul, a large, amiably shambling man with thinning hair and a constant expression of mild bemusement on his lugubrious features, was explaining to me one day how he had gone to visit a certain Lady Chesterton, a renowned character and eccentric who lived a few miles outside our village.

He rang the bell upon his arrival, and after a good five minutes waiting Lady Chesterton ambled into sight from the direction of the garden.

'Ah, good morning, vicar, how lovely to see you,' she said brightly. 'Would you care for a cup of tea?'

'Delighted,' murmured Paul unenthusiastically, having been subjected to Lady Chesterton's tea on a previous occasion. 'Absolutely delighted.'

'Splendid,' responded her ladyship. 'Do come in, vicar, please, do come in.'

So saying she led him into the impressive inner hall, muttering, 'Make yourself at home, vicar, please. Wander around as you like,' before disappearing through a door into the inner recesses of the building.

So Paul wandered around a bit as he liked, just as invited, admiring the numerous portraits of ancestral Chestertons adorning the walls and the newly refurbished stained glass window in the east wing. Somewhere in the stillness a clock chimed the half-hour, and then the three-quarters. Paul dutifully admired the pictures for a second time, and then started counting the number of black and white tiles on the entrance hall floor.

When the distant clock struck the hour he began to measure the hall's dimensions, walking pigeon-toed across the diagonals and making little notes on the back of his prayer book. Suddenly, as he was calculating exactly how many London taxis it would take to transport all the required tiles a distance of two hundred miles before breakfast, the front door flew open and in walked the good Lady Chesterton again, muttering furiously to herself.

Paul coughed discreetly, and she looked up, surprised.

'Oh, hello, vicar,' she said, even more brightly than before, 'how lovely to see you. Would you like a cup of tea?'

And it is not just me that forgets things in the surgery – patients have been known to transgress too. A university don of no more than late middle age sat before me once with that air of academic vagueness so characteristic of his species. Here was a man quite at home amongst Latin declensions incomprehensible to the rest of us, but completely incapable of managing the practicalities essential to a smooth-running existence. Simple things, such as taxing the car, for instance, using the TV remote control for any purpose other than scratching his ear, and managing to get the plastic toy out of the bottom of the cereal packet without spilling Coco pops all over the breakfast table.

'What can I do for you?' I enquired politely, as he was not one of our most regular attenders. Regular attenders (or PITAs, as we call them, and you'll have to think about that) may be greeted by anything from a superficially welcoming 'Blood pressure check, is it, Mavis?' (quick and thankfully not in the least bit messy) to a resigned 'I suppose it's your bowels again, is it, Mr Stanbury?'

The university don looked at me vaguely. 'I'm not all that sure, really,' he said in a surprised fashion, rather as if I had asked him what colour socks he had worn a week last Thursday. I decided to be a little more direct.

'What are you actually here for?' I asked, which threw him completely. He looked at me blankly, checked his watch and suddenly gasped, 'It's Tuesday, isn't it?'

'It is,' I agreed politely. 'Has been most of the morning.'

'Then I shouldn't be here at all,' he said desperately. 'I should be researching the life and times of Graham the Second of England in Exeter Public Library, right about now.'

'Graham the Second of England,' I mused reflectively. 'I can't say that I've ever heard of him.'

'Which is precisely why my research is so important,' he answered enthusiastically. 'The lost King of our Empire States – sorry,' and he dashed out of the surgery without another word.

Which left me thinking, really. What sort of man mistakes a small rural surgery for a library in a decent-sized city over forty miles away? What type of academic honestly believes we as a nation could ever crown a man with the unfortunate name of Graham?

And then the answer came to me. A man who reads Latin and Greek for fun.

As the crow flies, the farm on which Mary lived was no more than a couple of miles and a dirt track road or two away from the branch surgery.

But this is Devon, and Devon crows have no sense of direction . . .

Twenty minutes later I negotiated the last rut in the final lane and drew up into a typical farmhouse courtyard. Scattered around me, in no particular order, were arrayed a mud-spattered Land Rover or two, a couple of dogs – one chained and barking, and the other lying down by the kitchen window not bothering to bark at all – and a lost sheep munching phlegmatically at what used to be growing in the window box.

Sometimes there might be a hen or two, a duck or a handful of cows, but never a farmer. They are all off at market, or deep in conversation in the pub. As usual the thing you noticed first was the smell, whereas the last thing you noticed as you drove off . . . well, it was the smell, actually.

In between you get to deal with the reason you turned up in the first place, and my reason was in bed in a downstairs room looking yellow, and ill, and not very long for this world.

'Hello, Mary. How are you feeling?' I asked gently.

'Fine, thank you, Doctor,' she answered. 'How nice of you to come and see me. I'm just a little tired, maybe.'

'Any pain anywhere?'

'A little, doctor, but no more than I can deal with.'

I felt her stomach cautiously, noting the firmness in the top right-hand corner, and the wince she tried unsuccessfully to conceal when I pressed there.

'You're a little bit yellow, Mary, had you noticed?' I asked. Mary's daughter was standing just to one side, watching intently.

'Well, maybe a bit,' admitted Mary, and then she went quiet for a moment. You could almost hear the wheels turning, and then she said, 'A bit of my old trouble back again, do you think?'

'Yes, I think you are probably right,' I agreed.

'But it's not . . . is it . . . it's not . . . ?' she asked in trepidation.

'Not at all,' I interrupted. 'I'm sure it's not that at all.'

She lay back on her pillow and closed her eyes. 'Oh good, doctor, I'm so glad. I'm so lucky to be able to trust you.'

My eyes met her daughter's, and we both shrugged slightly.

I admitted Mary to hospital that day, where she had scans, X-rays and a whole host of blood tests before a minor operation in which a tube was inserted to part of her gall bladder. When she came out again a week and a half later she was still far from well, but at least she wasn't yellow any more. I had rung the consultant before she went in, and nobody, but nobody had mentioned the word 'cancer' whilst she was an in-patient, a tremendous feat of co-operation and understanding.

And then Mary came home again, and after an initial visit following her discharge I stayed well away. Like many country people Mary thought that if the doctor came to visit her at home then she must indeed be unwell, whereas if he stayed away then probably all was fine.

Now this may not be a purely country phenomenon, but the following sort of conversation is not unknown in our practice. There are not that many meeting places in our small village – the pub in the evening, outside the school at pick-up and drop-off times, and the post office/village shop which is where I most often encounter my patients outside the surgery premises.

'Hello, Mr Brown, haven't seen you for a long time. How are you?'

'Much better now, doctor, thank you.'

'Oh . . . ' Doctor thinks furiously, wondering what he may have missed and asks hesitantly, 'Have you been unwell, then?'

'Yes, doctor, for some time now,' continued Mr Brown.

More furious thinking. No, I was sure I hadn't seen him myself.

'So,' I ventured cautiously, 'Dr Harper's been looking after you, has he?'

'Oh no, doctor, I've been much too ill to come down to the surgery. I'm going to make an appointment with you tomorrow, now that I'm better.'

You do have to be so careful. I was at a dinner party once when a middle-aged lady of the blue rinse brigade greeted me conversationally with the words, 'Good evening, Dr Sparrow, how nice to see you again.'

'Hello, Mrs Wilson, haven't seen you for . . . it must be ages.'

'Yesterday morning,' she said, peering at me over the rim of her glasses. 'On your couch, as it happens, and in a less than entirely dignified position.'

Nine months later, Mary was gradually deteriorating but had had no major problems. Her daughter rang me one lunchtime.

'She's failing fast,' she said, 'but it's outpatients tomorrow, and she desperately wants to go. Can you do the usual?'

'Of course,' I agreed. 'Do you want me to come and see her?'

'No, Dr Sparrow, not just now. Two doctors in two days – she'll think she must be dying.' Bessie gave a small chuckle. 'And we can't have that now, can we?'

I was called out before surgery the next day, and didn't have the chance to put the call through to outpatients until a quarter to ten in the morning.

I should at this point explain that the outpatients in question takes place not at the major hospital in Plymouth, our nearest big city, but at the small GP-run district hospital in Launceston. Consultants and junior staff in various specialities travel the half-hour or so up from the city on a regular basis.

Mary's consultant was away on holiday, and his registrar ill for the day, so instead of a well-known friendly voice at the end of the phone I encountered a sharp-toned locum consultant who answered my call tersely. I explained the circumstances and asked for his help.

'You mean you want me to lie to a patient I have never previously met to perpetuate your six years to date of systematic falsification of the truth? In addition, you apparently expect me to tell her she is not suffering from a condition which she quite clearly is, and isn't going to be dying soon when even a first-year medical student could easily discern precisely the opposite?'

'Spot on,' I said. 'That's about the size of it.'

'Well, I won't do it,' he said angrily. 'It's unprofessional, un-ethical and lays you open to all sorts of litigation.'

'So covering your own back is more important than looking after the patient and their real needs?' I asked. 'This is the countryside, may I remind you. Patients don't sue here for pro-tecting their interests – '

'You GPs are all the same,' he interrupted disparagingly. 'You spend so much of the time making sure you look all caring and vocational that you forget the basics we were each and every one of us brought up on – truth and honesty at all times. It's a hard world we professionals have live in whilst you soft-headed woolly-minded liberals are playing God with your patients because it makes you feel all warm and comfortable inside.'

He put the phone down just before I unveiled my ever-enlarging vocabulary of expletives deleted upon him. 'We professionals' indeed . . . who on earth did he think he was?

Six years of doing the best we could for Mary, and it was all about to be thrown away at the last moment. I sat in my office for a moment, stunned. Her appointment was just under an hour away, and I had to stop her going at all costs. Feverishly I looked up the phone number of the farm, misdialled in my haste and then sat chewing my nails as the phone rang, and rang, and rang.

Just as I was about to give up in despair, somebody answered.

''Ello,' said a deep voice I recognized as belonging to Brian, Mary's youngest grandson and now a strapping seventeen-year-old pulling his full sixteen stone weight on the farm.

'Thank goodness,' I said in relief. 'It's Dr Sparrow here, Brian. Can I talk to your mum?'

'No,' said Brian, a man of few words.

'Brian, it's important, I need to talk to her.'

'She's not here,' he said. 'Left five minutes ago to take Gran to the hospital. Can I help?'

'No, thanks, Brian,' I said absently. 'I'll catch her later.'

I put the phone down and sank my head in my hands in disappointment. Too late. I would just have to accept it.

Katherine, my practice nurse, came in at this point, pushing a supermarket trolley as she looked to retrieve the odd bit of equipment I had borrowed from her treatment room in a fit of absent-mindedness.

'And what's up with you?' she asked. 'Banged your knee on

the desk again? Stock market crashed irretrievably? West Ham on the brink of relegation? Or is it something important?'

I explained briefly, and sat looking and feeling probably at least half as sorry for myself as I did for Mary. 'It's too late,' I said hopelessly. 'What can I possibly do now?'

'Well,' she said slowly, 'you can sit there wallowing in self-pity and do nothing at all, or you can go back to basics.'

I looked at her quizzically. 'Back to basics?'

'Back to basics,' repeated Katherine firmly. 'What would you have done if you were still a student? Sat back and let it all go on around you, or got off your backside and gone and done something about it? Is there any real life or spirit left in that tired old body of yours, or are you merely still pretending to be an actively useful member of the human race?'

Somewhere deep inside the recesses of my brain an idea was beginning to form.

'Improvise,' she continued. 'Call in a few favours. Cheat, lie and blackmail, if you have to. But do something, for goodness sake. Be a man, not a paltry excuse for a mouse.'

'No, tell me what you really think I should do,' I said, a smile beginning to form on my face.

Katherine walked across the room, stood in front of my desk and rested her hands on the top of it, peering down into my face.

'I do believe I can see a glimmer of intelligent life,' she said shrewdly. 'So now, are you going to continue to sit there like a poor imitation of a cabbage, or are you going to get up and do something about it?'

'Never much liked cabbage myself,' I grinned, and started moving.

Mary died peacefully at home a week later, and I called in to see her the day before. She was heavily jaundiced and very wasted, but as always beautifully cared for by her daughter, not a pressure sore in sight.

'She's fading so fast,' said Bessie sadly as she met me at the doorway. 'It won't be long now, I'm sure, but she might still recognize you.'

I went through into Mary's small but tidy downstairs bedroom where she was sleeping peacefully, a diamorphine syringe driver slowly feeding a regular supply of painkiller into her arm. She couldn't have looked more at ease. As Bessie and I stood murmuring quietly together at the end of the bed Mary suddenly opened her eyes, bright, watery oases in the middle of her lined and yellowing face.

'Is that you, Bessie?' she called. 'Is that you, dear? Who have you got with you?'

Bessie sat down on the side of the bed and gently took her hand. 'It's the doctor, Mum. Dr Sparrow. He just called in to see how you were doing.'

I moved forward and sat down too, taking Bessie's place for a moment. 'Hello, Mary,' I said. 'How are you today?'

'Is that you, doctor?' she asked, reaching out tentatively for my hand and then grasping it tightly.

'Yes, Mary, it's me,' I replied.

She closed her eyes briefly, and then opened them again, a hint of a smile forming at the corner of her mouth. 'I know why you're here, doctor. I expect you think I'm just a silly old woman, but I know when my time is due.'

She struggled to sit upright, grasped my hand again firmly and with surprising strength between both of hers, and looked directly at me.

'Just tell me one thing, doctor, and tell me the truth, this one last time. It's not cancer, is it?'

I thought of my old professor's words about never lying to your patients, and lies becoming a cancer of their own. I thought about the locum consultant's dismissive remarks about GPs playing at being God for motives of their own, and then I ignored it, ignored it all in favour of good, old-fashioned common sense.

'No, Mary,' I said as firmly and positively as I could, 'it's not cancer, I promise you that.'

She gave a small sigh of relief and sank back into her pillow, exhausted. 'I'm so glad,' she whispered, 'so glad. And so lucky to have a doctor I can trust.'

Mary slipped off into a deep sleep then, her hold on my hand gradually lessening until it slipped from her grasp altogether. I left the room thoughtfully and stood talking to Bessie for a few moments out in the courtyard.

'Well, Dr Sparrow,' she said mischievously, 'it's probably none of my business, but was there something a little bit odd going on at outpatients last week?'

'Odd, Bessie?' I asked innocently. 'What sort of "odd" did you mean?'

'It just seemed . . . a bit tense in there,' she said with a twinkle in her eye. 'There was only one doctor that I could see, and then suddenly there was lots of noise and he ran out of the building just as it was Mum's appointment, and then another man came in that I vaguely recognized – ever so young he was – and Mum saw him instead.'

'And everything was fine after that?'

'Oh, everything was completely fine. Mum didn't notice a thing, and he was so kind and reassuring.'

'Well, that's splendid then, Bessie,' I said. 'I'm glad it all went well,' and I climbed into my car, turned on the engine and wound down the window to bid her farewell.

'But it was strange . . . ' said Bessie, looking at me thoughtfully.

'Strange?' I repeated matter of factly.

'Yes, strange,' said Bessie, 'because Mrs Allen, you know, she lives next door but one to my daughter-in-law's brother, well, she said that you dashed out in the middle of your surgery on an emergency that morning, and I thought I saw your car up at the hospital just as we were going in . . . '

'Really?' I murmured.

' . . . but I didn't see you anywhere there, Dr Sparrow. Did I?'

I smiled at her and put the car into gear.

'No, Bessie,' I said. 'I don't believe you did.'

A few days later Christine, my receptionist, buzzed through at the end of morning surgery.

'There's a gentleman here to see you,' she said. 'He didn't give his name, but said I had to be sure to tell you that he was just back from holiday, he knows you will be keen to see him, and that I was to say "Lotus Esprit" to you. He says he is sure you will understand.'

'You had better send him in,' I said, my pulse quickening slightly.

A few minutes later my consulting-room door opened, and in walked Mary's consultant surgeon with a grave expression on his face.

'Ah, Dr Sparrow,' he said seriously. 'I thought perhaps we had better have a word, now I am back at the helm again.'

'Uhuh,' I said non-committally. 'A word.'

'Or two,' he continued soberly, 'perhaps even three or four.' He stretched out his feet and settled back in his chair. 'Coffee would be nice.'

I buzzed back to reception. 'Could we have two black coffees, please?'

'And biscuits,' added my visitor.

'And biscuits,' I confirmed, listening for a moment and then looking back at him. 'She says will custard creams be OK?'

'Fine,' he nodded. 'My favourites.'

Once coffee and biscuits had arrived, he continued with the reason for his visit.

'Came back a day early from holiday, I did,' he said through a mouthful of biscuit, 'and had rather an interesting talk with my locum, one Mr Gibson. Didn't meet him by any chance, did you?'

'No, not as such,' I said. 'I did speak to him on the phone, though.'

He pursed his lips. 'Yes, he said as much. He was a funny sort of chap, to be sure, but things seemed to be going quite smoothly until a certain outpatients session. He was going to put in an official complaint, but he wasn't quite sure what he was complaining about, or even a hundred per cent certain who, but looking down the list of patients he was seeing at the time, and knowing you of old . . .'

'Well,' I said, recognizing defeat when I finally met it, 'it was sort of like this . . .'

As soon as Katherine left my room I had sat for a moment or two, considering all the possible alternatives, and then picked up the phone. Ten minutes of cajoling, pleading, begging, arm-twisting and emotional blackmail later, everything was arranged. Sort of. All that was needed was a steady nerve, a considerable amount of luck and a total disregard for the potential consequences of failure.

I made my way out towards the office, glancing through the window into the waiting room – three-quarters full and restless, but no actual rioting as yet – and said in a quick aside to Christine, 'I'm just going out for a bit.'

She raised her eyes to the heavens. 'Not again. And the patients?'

'Oh, just tell them the usual,' I said unsympathetically. 'Off on a visit, outbreak of Black Death at the Harmsworths', earthquake rumbling near Grinnacombe Moor – any old lie will do. Just make it convincing. There's a bonus in it for you.'

'Which is?' she responded, somewhat unconvinced.

'You'll still have a job in the morning,' I replied sweetly, slipping out of the back door. Sneaking into my car I drove off down the bypass to the local hospital at full speed, parking unobtrusively round at the back where the first of my fellow conspirators was waiting, a small bag in his hand.

'Which one?' he asked in a relaxed fashion.

I pointed. 'Any problem?'

'None whatsoever,' he grinned. 'This one will be a pleasure. Two minutes at the most.'

My first phone call had been to Lesley, an old friend and the nurse in outpatients. 'The locum surgeon,' I said, 'I need to know. What car does he drive?'

'Been boasting about it all morning,' she said disgustedly. 'Roared up in a Lotus Esprit, his pride and joy. Horrid little man – keeps calling me "dearie" and trying to look down the front of my dress.'

'Good,' I said, ' because I could do with a little favour.'

We spoke for a minute or two and then she put me through to the male nurse in casualty, who ran through a range of emotions from horrified, to appalled, inquisitive and then positively enthusiastic.

Finally I rang 'Psycho', a thin weaselly-looking man in his mid-thirties whose real name had long been forgotten, probably even by himself, and who owed me a favour or two. Psycho's speciality was cars; cleaning, mending, valeting – and occasionally borrowing, when the need arose.

I watched him stroll casually up to the Esprit, pleasure written all over his face at both the sight of the car and the prospect of what he was about to do to it.

In a matter of seconds the door was open and the engine running, and he threw me a wave as I slipped on a cap and a pair of sunglasses and slid easily behind the wheel, grinning from ear to ear. This was going to be fun.

I drew slowly up to the back entrance of the hospital, the car purring ecstatically beneath me, and gave a quick toot on the horn. Lesley stuck her head out of the door, waved energetically and disappeared back inside again.

A matter of moments later an enraged locum consultant surgeon burst out into the car park, almost catching me by surprise, and threw himself at the car as just in the nick of time I let in the clutch and unleashed the Lotus like a caged lion. We shot down the drive together, Mr Gibson charging behind us in hot pursuit.

Back inside the hospital things were running smoothly to plan. Right on cue, Lesley had stuck her head around the surgeon's door and said breathlessly, 'I think somebody's stealing your car.'

Out ran he as anticipated, whilst ten seconds following his departure in strolled the young male nurse from casualty sporting a long white coat with a stethoscope draped carelessly round his neck, looking for all the world like the young high-flying surgeon he wasn't.

'Next patient if you will, please, sister,' he said lightly, settling himself into the surgeon's chair as if to the manner born. Lesley winked at him before crossing the few steps to the waiting room.

'Mary Smith,' she called. 'Doctor's ready for you now.'

Outside, I slowed down at the hospital entrance, for one heart-stopping moment almost stalling the engine. Unaccustomed to the car, I clashed gears and revved frantically, the ever-enlarging view of Mr Gibson looming ominously in the rear-view mirror. At the last moment I recovered my composure and began to edge slowly, enticingly towards the supermarket next door, with him now beginning to labour visibly in my wake.

One last final burst, a blissful surge on the throttle that I would sell my soul to have at my command each and every day, and I was round to the back of the building and out of sight for a few crucial minutes. Adrenaline coursing through my veins, I was out of the car, over the fence separating the car park from the back of the hospital, and in my own car on the way down the hospital drive just as the surgeon arrived at his now empty

Lotus Esprit where he stood, hands on knees, breathing heavily and wondering just what on earth was going on.

Lesley stuck her head out of the window as I cruised past on my way back to the surgery, giving me the thumbs up and smiling happily ...

'And that's it,' I said as I finished my explanation, spreading my arms and holding my palms out in front of me as Mary's surgeon sat back in his chair, pursing his lips and regarding me thoughtfully.

'Thought it might be something like that,' he mused. 'Now, let me get this right. What you're basically saying is that not only have you lied systematically and deliberately to a patient for the past six years about her medical condition, you have also stolen ... '

'Borrowed,' I put in, trying to sound emotionally distressed.

' ... stolen my locum's car and inveigled an innocent male nurse to impersonate a senior doctor. Is that about the size of it?'

I considered the matter carefully, and then 'Yup,' I agreed.

'Enough to have you struck off for the next couple of decades, in fact.'

'Yup.'

'I should report you.'

'Yup, I guess you should,' I shrugged.

'To every professional body I have ever heard of.' He sighed and shook his head in disbelief. 'So tell me, Dr Sparrow, do you have an explanation for all this, then?'

And I looked at him, and he looked at me, and then we both started grinning.

'I suppose,' said Declan O'Shaughnessy, my long-time friend and now incumbent consultant surgeon at the City General Hospital in Plymouth, 'you could say you were just ... '

' ... exercising my clinical judgement,' we finished together.

13

Walking the Tightrope

As I sit here in my back garden with a glass of wine in my hand, my newspaper waiting patiently on the table to be read, the smell of a recently smoked cigar hovering on the still evening air and the sound of my children screaming at the top of their voices over whatever their latest trivial disagreement has been, there is time at last to reflect upon the day, and the week, and the way that life now is.

It is always and ever my favourite part of the day. Work is over, for a start, and the stresses and stains – no, it's not a typing error – of the past twelve hours or so are melting into the faint mist on the horizon. The sun setting gently behind me floods the valley ahead with that familiarly beautiful, tranquil glow, and in the far distance the hills and tors of Dartmoor can be seen sinking slowly into the twilight.

This is my world. From my vantage point at the top of the hill I can see most of my practice area spread out before me, from Brentor Church standing proud upon its lonely hill fifteen miles south-west to the acrid-smelling smoke from the abattoir some twenty miles north. Within this compact hundred or so square miles the Mary Smiths, the Lady Chestertons, Sylvia and Jim's, not to mention so many more, have lived and toiled, been born and died, moved in and moved out of my life.

I wouldn't have missed a moment of it, for the world.

Right now, right at this moment I think I must I have everything I have ever wanted. A country practice in Devon and Cornwall, a house that owns my soul, a family I would die for –

but not just yet, if nobody minds – and a motley collection of pets with indiscriminate bowel habits.

Absolute heaven.

Yet it could have been so very different. The toss of a coin, the turn of a page, and one moment, for ever imprinted upon my mind, as I stood and stared at a small brown envelope in my hand, hardly daring to breathe . . .

Oh yes – and that bit about the criminal record.

Most people have their own individual response to the deleterious effects of alcohol.

Some, for example, will merely fall soundly asleep, whilst others may start singing loudly and vociferously without worrying too much about the words, or the tune. Many of the rest will be picking fights, or chasing unsuitable or unattainable women, and some of us will do all four, in a varying order of merit. Most worrying of all are those who decide to tell you their life history.

But me – I used to climb things. Happily, increasing age and infirmity have precluded this pastime from progressing into middle age. Lamp-posts were a favourite at the time – it may be hard to understand precisely why, but suffice it to say that when walking home from the seemingly endless succession of late night parties at Great Ormond Street Hospital nurses' home at three o'clock in the morning, lamp-posts, like Mount Everest, were just *there*.

Lamp-posts were duly superseded by drainpipes, and then scaffolding. Once, after a particularly bad night, I can vaguely recall scaling the dizzy heights of one of those monstrous cranes that used to suddenly appear in the back streets of Euston and King's Cross, lumbering through the concrete jungle like some giant alien Meccano dinosaur, looking for a quiet, secure place to rest for the night.

In my worst dreams, I imagine I am still up there . . .

I am convinced that climbing this last edifice was responsible for my present-day vertigo, which is bordering on the terminally pathetic. I felt particularly abject as I clung like a limpet to the central column at the top of the Eiffel Tower as if my life depended on it, whilst my children were running around the upper balcony calling out excitedly, 'Wow, Daddy, look at the view.' It is a touch difficult to admire the magnificently sweeping vista laid out below you if your eyes are tight shut, and in any case I knew, I just *knew,* that if a single gust of wind was ever going to blow the whole edifice over after 160 years or so of untroubled existence it was going to be right then, whilst I was at the top.

After a spot of medical student-orientated climbing it would be time to indulge another whim. For some reason, medical students have always had a great affection for, and affiliation with, street signs. So much so, in fact, that admire them as we do in their natural setting it remains to us a wholly insufficient reason for leaving them there.

Indeed, no matter how exquisitely suited they may seem to be whilst they remain impaled upon the brick-lined streets of London, they look even more splendidly at home when adorning the walls of our bedsits. It takes but a short leap of the imagination to then understand that on the odd occasion we would feel justifiably emboldened to borrow them – temporarily, of course (and yes, I know that twenty or more years may not seem to you to quite fall under the category of temporary, but all things are relative) – and take them home for a spell, so to enhance our daily well-being.

And if that wasn't excuse enough, there was the competition . . .

I have long since forgotten the precise figures, but the St Mary's Hospital Medical School all-time record for street sign misappropriation in any one night by two people working in tandem stood at something like twenty in a four-hour period. This, let's face it, represented a challenge of such stature and standing that no self-respecting student could fail to have at least one attempt to better it — especially at one o'clock in the morning when an impromptu party was in full swing.

November 1976, and on one such night we had all the requisite ingredients in place to launch a realistically attainable challenge. These comprised a large gathering of students, equal numbers of nurses too inexperienced to have yet started going out with doctors, lashings of cheap alcohol and soggy crisps, and somebody's stereo blasting out into the night keeping all the neighbours awake.

In the early hours of the morning my partner in crime, Peter (now Dr) Williams, and I stood looking solemnly at a collection of fifteen lovingly accumulated street signs in the corner of the room.

The record was on.

'One more trip should do it,' we agreed soberly — well, soberlyish — as the party continued to rock and roll uninhibitedly around us.

I seem to recall that some poor misguided fool did actually say, 'Why don't you stop while you're ahead? You're just asking for trouble . . .' which of course made us even more determined — or in other words more stupid — than before.

As there were now very few street signs in the immediate vicinity still attached to their original wall, and most of those were beyond our limited reach, we were obliged to forage further afield. Which is where our troubles really began, for suddenly we found ourselves standing outside the Royal Free Hospital Medical School.

That in itself would not normally have presented us with a problem, Peter and I having both been there before and survived the experience without incident. Sadly, however, on this occasion we were seized by an overriding impulse to be inside — rather than outside — the medical school, and, more specifically, inside the bar.

Now this was not what you might initially think.

This being the Royal Free, the bar would have long since been shut for the night, all the hot chocolate and Ovaltine having been consumed and the Free-ites having retired to their beds. But we knew that in the aforementioned bar there proudly reposed a sign most evilly stolen from our own medical school some years before by an enterprising Royal Free student – probably the only one they have ever had.

It was not even that it was a particularly grand sign, and nor was it in itself of any great historical significance. It wasn't even especially aesthetically pleasing, being wooden, badly scratched and in need of several new coats of varnish.

But it was there, and it was ours, and it said 'St Mary's Hospital' on it.

We stood and looked at each other, and said with one voice, 'The time has come to go and get it back.'

Progressing from the outside of the building to the 'in' proved to be a bit of a problem. Not entirely to our surprise – this being three o'clock in the morning – the front door was shut, and there was not the merest hint of a friendly night-watchman to let us in. The rest of the ground floor was a complete non-starter, but this being an old London building it had a basement and a below-ground walkway that extended three-quarters of the way round, ending in a blind alley. We clambered over a locked iron gate ineffectually guarding the entrance and descended some concrete steps into the basement area, walking its full length before coming out again, having found no obvious point of access.

We were on the point of giving up when inspiration struck. To our left was a conveniently situated drainpipe, and above our heads a partly open third-floor window. It was a heaven-sent opportunity.

I started climbing . . .

Five minutes later I had made my way back down to the basement, opening a door at one end of the blind alley to let Peter in to join me, drainpipe climbing not being one of his favourite pastimes.

Twenty minutes of happy wandering through a dark and silent

medical school later, with our newly reclaimed sign now firmly in our grasp, we decided it was time to make our way back to the party, which we were in no doubt would still be merrily continuing despite our extended absence. We slipped out again through the same basement door we had entered, closing it firmly shut behind us (a great mistake, this, as events were subsequently to prove) and passed back round the alley to the steps up to the iron railings at street level . . . which is where we stopped, stone dead, and open-mouthed in horror.

Three Black Marias (a little bit like old Ford Transit vans, for those of you too young to remember) and four or five police cars were parked at the end of the cordoned-off street. Half a dozen police officers were milling around ominously, and a couple of very large police dogs were tugging ferociously at their chains, salivating away, no doubt looking forward to a juicy limb or two to sink their teeth into.

'Can't be here for us,' I murmured unconvincingly. 'Can they?'

'Can't be,' agreed Peter, equally hesitantly. 'But just to be on the safe side . . .'

We retreated rapidly back into the basement area and returned to our point of exit from the building, where the door remained steadfastly closed despite our best efforts to reopen it. Fumbling around in the dark we could feel – apart from an awful lot of wall – some sort of redundant machinery, which seemed probably to be an old generator.

And then we sat and hid behind it, waiting for them all to go away. Because they couldn't, they just couldn't be there for us, could they, not all those vehicles, and policemen, and dogs . . ?

After a few minutes we heard footsteps in the street above us, and a torch flashed down briefly a few yards to the left of where we stood cowering motionless to the rear of the generator, hardly daring to breathe.

'See anything down there?' called one policeman to another.

'Blind alley and a door,' came the answer. 'Looks closed to

288

me,' and we relaxed momentarily until the second voice continued 'but you'd better take the dog down there and check it out. They've got to be around here somewhere.'

I think it was the word 'dog' that we found most worrying, as 'worrying' was what we imagined it to be doing to our legs in the very near future. Suddenly we were no longer in the jolly throes of an innocent student prank, but had been tipped headlong into something altogether more serious.

'What shall we do now?' hissed Peter nervously in my ear.

'Panic,' I suggested practically, 'and start thinking of an alternative career . . . '

A few moments later a policeman duly came round the corner of the alley and walked down to the cul-de-sac where we stood huddled together – but sadly he was not alone. Pulling hard at his choke chain was an awful lot of police dog with a hungry look about him, as if he had left for work without breakfast and was just ready for some late night refreshment.

Now I have no rational explanation for what happened next, but I swear to you it is completely true. The policeman drew to a halt within a foot of where we stood and peered around in the dark, obviously unable to see anything at all.

'What's down there?' called the voice from above.

'Oh, just old machinery of some sort,' came the reply, so close to my ear that I wondered if we were in the presence of a brand new initiative in the Met, 'Blind Policemen and Guide Dogs on the Beat – is This the Way Forward?' As this incongruous idea was still running through my head he kicked first the nearest iron stanchion and then Peter's shin (I shared his pain, figuratively speaking) with his heavily shod boot.

Somehow, amazingly, Peter managed to move not a fraction of an inch, and avoided all involuntary yelps. It was clear that the policeman had no idea at all of our presence in his immediate vicinity.

But the bit I cannot explain to this day is the behaviour of the dog. He snuffled around for a few moments in the corners, wagging his tail amiably, gave my hand a quick lick and then ambled off insouciantly with his disappointed handler in tow.

'Nobody down 'ere, John,' he called up to his colleague. 'Bit of a wild goose chase, if you ask me.'

It was really quite staggering. All those police vehicles and searching officers, not to mention being eyeball to eyeball with both dog and handler, and we had remained undiscovered. The relief was overwhelming.

'A miracle is born,' I whispered to Peter, but unfortunately for us it died as quickly as it had emerged, blinking, into the light. Another policeman above us threw down a torch to a second policeman below – without dog, this one – who walked back along to our cul-de-sac and shone his light through the door opposite us into the room beyond, equally unaware of our presence behind him.

''E's right,' he declared positively, turning to walk finally away, 'there's nothing down here but a whole load of rubbish.'

Our totally undeserved freedom was all but guaranteed . . . until the torch, hanging loosely in his hand, swung its beam crazily around the wall as he turned to go, catching our startled and aghast faces fairly and squarely in its unremitting glare.

'Evening, officer,' I said politely. 'Nice night for a stroll.'

'Cor,' he responded in complete surprise, 'where the bloody 'ell did you two spring from, then?' as if impressed by our Houdini-like appearance on the scene.

I was just about to enter into a metaphysical discussion on the point when he suddenly remembered that he was a member of the Metropolitan Police Force, and we were the fugitives that he, his colleague and his colleague's dog had all failed initially to spot. Things spiralled downhill from this point.

It's quite an experience, travelling in the back of a Black Maria, but not one I would necessarily recommend. Nor, if I'm honest, is sitting cold and alone in a police cell in Central London having just been arrested for breaking and entering.

There is, I put it to you, something inherently amiss in the criminal justice system, as there was not then – and I believe still is not now – a category of offence known as 'Harmless medical student misdemeanours', or 'Meaninglessly drunken theft of big things you don't need'. This latter one, in particular, would come in very handy when you woke up and found a four-foot plastic ice-cream cone unexpectedly in your bedroom, or an authentic red telephone box in the hall of residence foyer, which, to this day, given the appalling difficulty we had trying to get it out again, I have not the least idea how we got in, in the first place.

Even more worryingly, there is as yet no known punishment like, for instance, 'Having a really good laugh about it, and then letting you go home'.

Consequently I sat – not, I am ashamed to say, for the first time in my life, nor even the last – contemplating the end of my career before it had even started. It was then five days short of the end of the autumn term in our second year, a small matter of three and a half years to go. Or at least it had been until that night, from which three and a half days might have been a better estimate.

Peter, I have to say, if contemplating anything at all, was doing so entirely unconsciously, if the sound of the snores emanating from the cell next to me were anything to go by. Certainly the gentle encouragement of our captors – 'Oy, you there, wake up mate,' – was proving to be ineffective, maybe the amount of alcohol consumed during the evening's festivities being a moderately relevant factor.

I was not lonely for long.

Two rather large gentlemen from the Metropolitan Police Force – who appeared to have had their senses of humour expertly excised by a very talented neurosurgeon – came to talk to me about crime in general, and how medical students in particular could no longer expect to get away with anything short of manslaughter just because we were lovable chaps with our hearts in the right places even if our bodies should prove to be in the wrong ones.

There then followed what I think can best be described as a full and frank exchange of views, during which I endeavoured to persuade them that having found myself – greatly to my surprise – thirty feet up a drainpipe I had duly panicked and taken the nearest escape route available. This, under the circumstances, happened to be the fortuitously open third-floor window at the Royal Free Medical School, and wasn't it lucky it was there just when I needed it. (I learned from their subsequent response that someone had actually seen me climbing in through it and dialled 999, which explained our over-enthusiastic reception party.)

Trying to convince them that this wholly innocent behaviour was neither a criminal offence nor worthy of their no doubt valuable time was proving to be a bit of a struggle. On reflection I was probably talking us into more trouble than I was delivering us out of when relief appeared in the shape of a senior policeman who opened the door and said tersely to my kindly interrogators, 'OK, you two – you're wanted elsewhere. I'm sure Mr Big here will keep for another hour or two.'

They arose to depart with ill-disguised bad grace, and shortly afterwards Peter and I were ejected unceremoniously into the streets of Bloomsbury, bleary-eyed, hungover and unshaven, as dawn was breaking over the horizon. The city slept on, unaware of – and no doubt uninterested in – two crestfallen medical students just beginning to come to terms with the predicament in which they had landed themselves.

Four days later we sat in the pub across the road from the medical school with the bulk of the rest of our year. It was lunchtime, and the last day of term.

Peter and I had of course been impeccably behaved in the interim, apart from the small matter of my waking him up on a park bench that morning. This would have been distinctly less disconcerting had the bench still been in Hyde Park, where it belonged, and not in fact in Peter's room in the hall of residence some three-quarters of a mile away.

'How on earth did you get it here?' I asked, both impressed and appalled at one and the same time.

'Carried it,' he said carelessly, as if it had been his shopping from Tesco's. 'Under cover of darkness.'

'Why, for God's sake?' I asked. 'You must be mad. And on the very night before we are up in front of our panel of executioners?'

'Same reason Edmund Hillary climbed Mount Everest,' he shrugged. 'Same reason you stole that telephone box from Sussex Gardens. One, because it was there, and two, because you seized that window of opportunity. There is a slide . . . '

'I think you mean tide,' I corrected him kindly.

' . . . in the affairs of men, and all that. The impending prospect of our imminent expulsion from the medical school is a mere irrelevance. The bench may not have been there tomorrow, nor I,' added Peter with a catch in his voice, becoming misty-eyed, 'here to pinch it.'

There was a logic in there that I could fully understand, not to mention the overriding reason for us doing anything at all of this nature, which is almost too obvious to mention.

Because it seemed like a good idea at the time.

As we sat there in the pub, an array of drinks in front of us courtesy of the well-wishers in our co-existent year, we had just emerged from our second full and frank exchange of views in far too short a timespan for my liking. The panel of executioners had consisted of the Dean, the Professor of Surgery – not my number one fan, in fact not even in the top twenty – and the senior Professor of Anatomy. A bit like the Holy Trinity, I suppose, but with a hell of a lot more bite.

Watching them at work, if you could detach yourself from the fact that it was us they were working upon, was really rather an interesting experience. The Professor of Surgery, who had no specific axe to grind save for his abhorrence of pre-clinical students in general and myself in particular, was using a lot of phrases along the lines of 'grossly irresponsible', 'reprehensible behaviour' and more worryingly, 'must make an example of them', coupled with 'expelled if I had my way'.

The man was obviously deranged, and big time.

The Professor of Anatomy, however, was without a shred of doubt a well-adjusted philanthrope who could actually recall being a student himself and would intersperse at regular intervals in tones of some awe, 'You had had *how* much to drink?', 'You climbed *how* high up the drainpipe?' and 'You say there was a sign of *ours*, actually in their *bar*?'

The Dean, a man of few words but most of them uncomplimentary, sat between them looking for all the world like a tennis umpire during a match full of especially long base-line rallies.

As all of us in that room knew, the tide was beginning to turn in the 'Medical Students v. the Rest of the World' debate. No longer could we be guaranteed to escape the consequences of our downright irresponsible behaviour, as we had so easily in the past. A sense of responsibility was slowly creeping into the system, and we were there to be made an example of, a lesson for our legion of successors to learn from.

And yet I would contend that we weren't such terribly awful people, not really – ringing our mothers at least once every term, helping old ladies across the road, whether they wanted to go or not . . .

So the Dean was caught, between the 'Hang 'em and flog 'em' attitude of the Professor of Surgery, and the gently shrugging shoulders and 'Boys will be boys' approach of that nice Professor of Anatomy. And Peter and I were caught too, and for once there was nothing either of us could do about it . . .

He kept us waiting, too, the swine.

For the first fortnight of the Christmas holiday I was up at the crack of each dawn, prowling the streets in search of the postman lest my parents should spot the fateful letter before I could retrieve it surreptitiously from the mat. On the fifteenth day I overslept, awaking to find my father standing by my bedside holding an official-looking brown envelope.

'It's marked "Private and Confidential", ' he said mildly. 'I take it this is the one you've been waiting for.'

I nodded, unable to trust myself to speak.

'Then I will leave the two of you alone together to become better acquainted,' he said, withdrawing to the door and then turning back for a moment.

'Of course,' he added drily, 'I have no idea what this letter is about, but I have not been your father for the past nineteen years without gleaning some basic understanding of the sort of person you are. Neither am I completely unaware of how medical students spend what passes as their leisure hours. And if on the basis of what you are waiting so desperately to read the minute I have left your room you were to be thrown out of that noble establishment, just consider what a favour you would be doing me.'

'A favour?' I said, momentarily confused.

'Yes, a favour,' he repeated, smiling not unkindly. 'Think of the money I would be saving on your grant.'

I have the letter still, and every once in a while I read it to remind myself of how thin the line can be between success and abject failure.

This chapter, I should add, was the last my mother read before her death on 5 August 2001, after a short illness.

'Ah,' she said, handing it back to me with a sigh. 'Do you know, I'd always wondered what that letter was about . . . '

It was in the balance. The Dean, having heard from all sides, brought the hearing to a close with one final question.

'So tell me honestly,' he had said, 'and I shall know if you are lying to me. Was this . . . jaunt of yours a pre-meditated act, or just a spur of the moment decision?'

'What did you say?' asked one of the students in the bar.

'Honesty is the best policy,' I said virtuously, 'so I looked him squarely in the eyes and said firmly, and with purity of heart, 'Completely spur of the moment, sir. We were just passing the medical school, spotted the open window and thought this would be a golden opportunity to reclaim part of Mary's pride and heritage, with no harm done to anyone. If only we had thought ahead and realized how much trouble we would be causing . . . ' I finished dolefully.

As I was repeating this to our audience in the pub, with not a little feeling, a thought struck me like a thunderbolt. I reached forward, tapped Peter on the shoulder and said urgently, 'Finish your drink, and come with me. I've just remembered something.'

'What?' he asked, irritated. 'I'm just beginning to enjoy myself here.'

'That alley where we were arrested – we've got to go back there,' I insisted.

'What the bloody hell for?' he asked, reaching for one of the three pints he had lined up in front of him.

'I've just remembered what I did with the sign,' I said pointedly.

'You mean . . ?' A look of horror began to dawn across his features.

'Yup,' I continued determinedly, 'I shoved it down behind the back of the generator, together with the hammer, the chisel, the jemmy and the complete set of adaptable screwdrivers . . . '